Praise for *The Mindful Me Journey*

"If you are interested in tackling your eating and exercise battles once and for all, this is the program for you! We all know how to step into the ostracizing or food eliminating rules of dieting and exercise, this workbook will kindly show you how to come to peace with your struggles and reside in your dreams. Do you want a step-by-step "walk home" to acceptance, love, self-care, and freedom from body or weight obsession? This is the journey for you!"

— Katie Hoffman, CMBB, CSMC
President, Stress Less Workshops

"This program guides individuals as they seek to revamp their relationship with nutrition and activity. Each journey is unique and so is this program. *The Mindful Me Journey* offers self-reflection in small steps that can be walked alone or with specialists in medicine and Medical Nutrition Therapy. As a Registered Dietitian, I would utilize this journaling program with a variety of individuals who have difficulty changing their health habits to maximize well-being."

— Lisa Sorn MS, RD, CSR, LD
Clinical Dietitian

THE MINDFUL ME JOURNEY

A 40-Day Guided Journal Toward a Healthier Relationship with Food and Exercise

THE MINDFUL ME JOURNEY

A 40-Day Guided Journal Toward a Healthier Relationship with Food and Exercise

TANYA FASNACHT JOLLIFFE, RDN, LD

THE MINDFUL ME JOURNEY
A 40-Day Guided Journal Toward a Healthier Relationship with Food and Exercise

Copyright © 2019 by Tanya Fasnacht Jolliffe, RDN, LD

All rights reserved. No part of this publication may be reproduced, stored in a retrieval system, or transmitted by any means—electronic, mechanical, photographic (photocopying), recording, or otherwise—without prior permission in writing from the author.

ISBN: 978-0-578-58180-4

Support: Rae Lynn DeAngelis and Melody Vanosdol Moore
Author photo credit: Don Denney and Mount St. Joseph University

Printed in the United States of America

First printing edition 2019

Learn more information at:
www.litwellnesssolutions.com

Disclaimer

The services provided through this self-reflection journaling program are not a substitute for medical, psychological, or dietetic care. This self-reflection journaling program is intended for use as a supplement to professional care and not as a replacement. It is your responsibility to obtain additional support through available resources. This program is best suited for someone in the rehabilitation or recovery stage.

This self-reflection journaling program may be used individually or with a professional counselor, medical, psychological, or dietetic professional. The activities in this book can be used as tools for discussion in a one-on-one or group settings. This program does not come with a guarantee and no direct counseling is provided to you through this self-reflection process or by the author.

This journaling program fits well as a follow-up to the Eyes Wide Open Healing Program by Living in Truth Ministries. Visit www.LivingInTruthMinistries.com to learn more.

Acknowledgments

To my parents, husband, children, family, coaches, teammates, co-workers, bosses, pastors, and church family. Thank you for traveling the road of life with me. Without all of you, I would not be the person I am today and this project would never have been possible. Praise and honor to the triune God that enables me to do exceedingly more through Him than I could ever accomplish on my own!

Table of Contents

Why Be Mindful? 1

Are You Ready to Get Started? 3

How to Use This Journal 5

Six Steps of Mindful Food and Exercise Change 7

Phase One: Exploring What You Are Doing and Why 9

Phase One Session Log Sheet (Day 1–10) 13

Phase One Reflection 93

Phase Two: Out with the Old, In with the New 97

Phase Two Session Log Sheet (Day 11–20) 99

Phase Two Reflection 179

Phase Three: Beginning to Build an Individualized Plan 183

Phase Three Session Log Sheet (Day 21–30) 187

Phase Three Reflection 267

Phase Four: Living a Nourishing and Active Life 271

Phase Four Session Log Sheet (Day 31–40) 275

Phase Four Reflection 315

Wrapping Up 317

Appendix 319

About the Author 329

Why Be Mindful?

We are each born with innate tendencies. Babies indicate when they are hungry and when they are full. Parents find it difficult sometimes to understand an infant's communication style. But make no mistake, babies know and communicate needs. Unfortunately, many of us have lost touch with those innate cues over the course of our lifetime. We can learn to get back in touch with our body and those innate cues through mindfulness.

Becoming mindfully aware of *what* we do and *why* we do it can help us unlock the chains that are holding us captive to disordered practices related to food and exercise.

Some examples might include:

- Learning to take notice of feelings of hunger and acting on them to nourish our body
- Noticing when we are full by slowing down the pace that we eat
- Noting when exercise is extreme and being used for reasons other than health
- Understanding that food is being selected to cope with emotions and feelings instead of finding another option
- Learning to make cognitive choices instead of continuing reactive habits

Once we have become mindfully aware of the habits, rules, routines, and rituals we have been following, we can move beyond them. That's what this next 40 days is all about.

Are You Ready to Get Started?

We are each an experiment of one. Our genetics, life experiences, habits, and tendencies are unique to us and like no one else. The journey taken that brought us to this point is equally as unique. The hurts, disappointments, and emotional/physical scars we bring are ours and no one else's. Many times those hurts and disappointments came because of other people who were carrying around their own emotional/physical scars. As the Will Bowen quote goes, "hurt people, hurt people."

The journey over the next 40 days will also be unique. There is no "one size fits all" approach that will break the chains holding you captive to chronic dieting or disordered eating and exercise. There ARE small, yet specific, mindful steps that you can take related to your habits and routines to set your feet firmly on a new path.

Are you willing to do the hard work necessary to honestly examine each and every food and exercise habit, feeling, and behavior you have? Are you willing to be mindfully present to face the food and exercise issues head on, so you can find a new way to relate to food and exercise? If so, the next 40 days you spend on a mindfulness path related to your eating and exercise can help you find freedom from the bondage of chronic dieting or disordered eating and exercise—FOREVER!

How to Use This Journal

This is a self-reflection journaling program designed to lead you through the process of becoming aware of thoughts, feelings, habits, and behaviors related to food and exercise. The first ten days are designed to be an "exploration phase." This phase will provide questions and prompts to help you learn how to be mindful of the thoughts, feelings, and behaviors you follow regarding food and exercise. As you move through the next ten days, you will be encouraged to begin to mindfully trade the negative and/or destructive decisions and activities for more positive alternatives.

The final twenty days on your mindfulness journey will focus on developing healthful eating and activity guidelines and guardrails. You will be coached to take small steps forward. You will be encouraged to accept a setback as just that, a step back that can be turned around tomorrow. You will begin to put mindful eating and activity practices into daily planning. You will mindfully process what you are doing and why you are doing it.

Let's be clear and honest. YOU are making unhealthy choices. This means YOU have the power and ability to make different choices, healthy choices, life giving and life sustaining choices. Self-reflection brings feelings and emotions into awareness. Through journaling, you will better understand the impact those feelings and emotions have on the food and/or exercise choices you make. In processing the "what" and "why" of your choices, you will likely face the internal critical voice that has been telling you WHO you are. This internal critic has been setting rules, placing compliance demands, and being overly critical of how you look and adhere to the rules and rituals. This voice may sound like a parent, coach, friend, or the media to you. Regardless of how this internal critic was formed, you have to recognize its power and shut it off to break its chains of control. You have to stop the lies of the negative voice and replace it with truth. This truth will take away the power the internal critic has had in your life.

You may also have to face:

- The reality that food or exercise is being used as a method of coping with unresolved feelings and issues related to a person or situation,
- How those unresolved feelings are being expressed through manipulated food and/or exercise,
- Understanding that they are reactions and responses that could be converted into alternative choices.

These next forty days provide you with a wonderful opportunity. You have an opportunity to express the emotion and pain through words. The opportunity to experience the process of turning them into constructive choices instead of manipulated food or exercise habits, rituals, routines, and behaviors. It is time to recognize and work through those painful feelings. Time to find a new capacity for self-regulation and expression that doesn't come through manipulated food or exercise. It is time to break the chains that have been holding you captive, time to nurture your body, mind, and spirit to live a healthy, happy, and whole life!

Six Steps of Mindful Food and Exercise Change

Review and agree to these six steps of mindful change and take the first step toward breaking free from food and exercise strongholds.

1. I admit that I am powerless over food and/or exercise and my life has been unmanageable.
2. I believe that a Power greater than myself can restore me to sensible eating and exercise.
3. I will fearlessly search my food and exercise habits and behaviors as expressions of my emotions, hurts, and disappointments.
4. I have or will admit to God, myself, and to another human being the exact nature of my disordered eating and/or exercise.
5. I will continually take a mindfulness inventory of my eating and exercise behavior and when they are unsound, I will promptly admit it.
6. Having had a spiritual awakening and mindful awareness of my food and exercise behavior, I will try to carry the message of mindful eating and exercise forward and to practice the principles in all my food and exercise habits.

Phase One

Exploring What You Are Doing and Why

What is 'normal' when it comes to eating and exercise? The dictionary provides a definition of normal as "conforming to a standard; usual, typical, or expected."[1] For many people, chronic dieting, disordered habits, and unhealthy routines have become normal. Our first step in breaking the chains of food and exercise strongholds is to identify *your* normal.

Let's start by establishing some common understanding related to the areas you will be addressing in the days ahead.

- **Self-image** - How you value yourself in relationship to food, exercise, and health habits. How your self-image influences your choices, selections, self-talk, and rationalizations related to the choices made.
- **Self-discipline** - Your willingness to exert self-control when making food, exercise, and health choices. Does your self-discipline improve your health or keep you in bondage?
- **Emotions** - Your ability to cope with emotional reactions and identify when they interfere with judgements related to consistency and quality of food and exercise choices.
- **Feelings** - How you recognize and subjectively respond to your emotions and how they influence your food and exercise decisions.

---

1. "normal". OED Online. September 2019. Oxford University Press. http://www.oed.com/viewdictionaryentry/Entry/11125 (accessed September 30, 2019).

- **Time** - How you manage your time in relation to food, exercise, work, family, and social interactions.
- **Other people** - Are you able to cope effectively and assertively with other people related to their expectations and values compared to your own?
- **Events** - How well do you balance and adjust eating and exercise patterns related to situations that take you away from your usual routine and plans?

In this first phase of your journey, you will be taking a closer look at what you are doing and why you are doing it. Changing unhealthy habits into nourishing ones is not easy. There are always setbacks and hard days. Learning to recognize what is going on and why it is happening allows you to adjust. Let's get started learning why we make some of the choices we do.

During the next ten days, you will complete a session log for *each* food or exercise related activity you undertake. You will log the basic information of the date, time, and reason for the session. *Session* is simply what you are doing whether that is eating a meal, having a snack, or taking a walk. Below that, you will note the specifics about the session, such as the reason for your session. Then you will reflect on the emotions and feelings you experienced before, during, and after the session.

The final part of the journaling experience for each session is to reflect on the activity and the emotions related to the choices made. You will note there is no specific journaling of food. You should address what you ate or how you exercised in the journaling reflection area. The "why" behind the "what" is key to this portion of your journey. If you had specific rules you followed when eating or certain expectations surrounding your activity, journal about them. If you need more space to journal than is provided, use a separate notebook for the additional space needed.

Ideally you will use a *new entry* for each session. The more focused you become about each session, the more you can identify what you are doing and why. If you do not have the time to commit to that level of discovery, doing one entry at the end of the day that captures the highlights is also an option. However, you will get more from this experience if you put in the time necessary to unpack what it going on and why. If you run out of session journal entry space before your last session on day 10, please go to the appendix section of the journal and make additional copies. If you get to your last session of day 10 and you aren't at the end of the provided Phase One journaling pages, move on to the Phase One Reflection activity. Once you have completed your last session on day 10, take some time to complete the *Phase One Reflection* questions. In this journaling activity you will look back at what you did and take a deeper look at the why of the patterns and choices you made. This self-reflection will prepare you for the next ten days of phase two. Be sure to allow time to reflect and journal after *each* session as well as at the end of day 10. This introspection and self-examination is the key to the locks that hold the chains that bind you to chronic dieting or total disorder.

PHASE ONE SESSION LOG SHEET

Day 1 - Day 10

Day 1

Complete the log for this food/exercise session. Place a checkmark next to or circle all that apply.

Date: 8-7-23   **Day of Week:** Monday   **Time:** 9 (AM)/PM

Reason for the session: (Meal)   Snack   Exercise   Other (Explain)

Who joined you: **Or Circle:**   (Ate Alone)/Exercised Alone

Did you count calories eaten or expended? Yes (No) **Why?**

Meal/Snack location:

(Dining Table)   Restaurant   In front of TV/Computer
In bed   Automobile   Other (Explain)

Beverage Consumed:

Soda   Diet soda/seltzer water   Tap/bottled water
Milk/dairy alternative   Other (Explain) Coffee

Reason for Eating:

(Nourishment)   Health   Social Activity/Group Gathering
Coping with feelings   Controlling Emotions   Other (Explain) HABIT

Reason for Exercise: (Check or circle the major reasons)

Appearance/Weight Maintenance   Fitness/Health Management
Stress/Emotions/Mood or Feeling Management   Socializing
Gardening

At the beginning, during, or conclusion of the meal/snack/exercise, I felt: (Circle all that apply to any phase of this session)

Bad	Numb	Panic	Empowered	Distressed	Successful
Worried	Anxious	Sad	Depressed	Relief	Motivated
Fear	Lonely	Angry	Contempt	Calm	Self-Disciplined
Comfort	Misery	Control	Driven	Soothed	Traumatized
Shame	Guilt	Tired	Hungry	Other (List)	

ACTIVITY REFLECTION

Journal some thoughts about the meal or snack you selected or the exercise you undertook. Why did you select what you did? How did the choices relate to the rules, habits, and rituals your internal critic helped you set up?

EMOTION REFLECTION

Journal about how the activity reflected the emotions you identified that went along with the activity. What brought the feelings/emotions on? Did they change during the session? What helped them change? Why did you select food/exercise as an outlet for those feelings?

When you complete your last session of Day 10, move on to the Phase One Reflection.

Phase One Session Log Sheet

Day 1 - Day 10

Complete the log for this food/exercise session. Place a checkmark next to or circle all that apply.

Date: **Day of Week:** **Time:** AM/PM

Reason for the session: Meal Snack Exercise Other (Explain)

Who joined you: **Or Circle:** Ate Alone/Exercised Alone

Did you count calories eaten or expended? Yes No **Why?**

Meal/Snack location:

Dining Table	Restaurant	In front of TV/Computer
In bed	Automobile	Other (Explain)

Beverage Consumed:

Soda	Diet soda/seltzer water	Tap/bottled water
Milk/dairy alternative	Other (Explain)	

Reason for Eating:

Nourishment	Health	Social Activity/Group Gathering
Coping with feelings	Controlling Emotions	Other (Explain)

Reason for Exercise: (Check or circle the major reasons)

Appearance/Weight Maintenance	Fitness/Health Management
Stress/Emotions/Mood or Feeling Management	Socializing

At the beginning, during, or conclusion of the meal/snack/exercise, I felt: (Circle all that apply to any phase of this session)

Bad	Numb	Panic	Empowered	Distressed	Successful
Worried	Anxious	Sad	Depressed	Relief	Motivated
Fear	Lonely	Angry	Contempt	Calm	Self-Disciplined
Comfort	Misery	Control	Driven	Soothed	Traumatized
Shame	Guilt	Tired	Hungry	Other (List)	

ACTIVITY REFLECTION

Journal some thoughts about the meal or snack you selected or the exercise you undertook. Why did you select what you did? How did the choices relate to the rules, habits, and rituals your internal critic helped you set up?

EMOTION REFLECTION

Journal about how the activity reflected the emotions you identified that went along with the activity. What brought the feelings/emotions on? Did they change during the session? What helped them change? Why did you select food/exercise as an outlet for those feelings?

When you complete your last session of Day 10, move on to the Phase One Reflection.

Phase One Session Log Sheet

Day 1 - Day 10

Complete the log for this food/exercise session. Place a checkmark next to or circle all that apply.

Date: **Day of Week:** **Time:** AM/PM

Reason for the session: Meal   Snack   Exercise   Other (Explain)

Who joined you: **Or Circle:**   Ate Alone/Exercised Alone

Did you count calories eaten or expended? Yes   No   **Why?**

Meal/Snack location:

Dining Table	Restaurant	In front of TV/Computer
In bed	Automobile	Other (Explain)

Beverage Consumed:

Soda	Diet soda/seltzer water	Tap/bottled water
Milk/dairy alternative	Other (Explain)	

Reason for Eating:

Nourishment	Health	Social Activity/Group Gathering
Coping with feelings	Controlling Emotions	Other (Explain)

Reason for Exercise: (Check or circle the major reasons)

Appearance/Weight Maintenance	Fitness/Health Management
Stress/Emotions/Mood or Feeling Management	Socializing

At the beginning, during, or conclusion of the meal/snack/exercise, I felt: (Circle all that apply to any phase of this session)

Bad	Numb	Panic	Empowered	Distressed	Successful
Worried	Anxious	Sad	Depressed	Relief	Motivated
Fear	Lonely	Angry	Contempt	Calm	Self-Disciplined
Comfort	Misery	Control	Driven	Soothed	Traumatized
Shame	Guilt	Tired	Hungry	Other (List)	

ACTIVITY REFLECTION

Journal some thoughts about the meal or snack you selected or the exercise you undertook. Why did you select what you did? How did the choices relate to the rules, habits, and rituals your internal critic helped you set up?

EMOTION REFLECTION

Journal about how the activity reflected the emotions you identified that went along with the activity. What brought the feelings/emotions on? Did they change during the session? What helped them change? Why did you select food/exercise as an outlet for those feelings?

When you complete your last session of Day 10, move on to the Phase One Reflection.

Phase One Session Log Sheet

Day 1 - Day 10

Complete the log for this food/exercise session. Place a checkmark next to or circle all that apply.

Date: **Day of Week:** **Time:** AM/PM

Reason for the session: Meal Snack Exercise Other (Explain)

Who joined you: **Or Circle:** Ate Alone/Exercised Alone

Did you count calories eaten or expended? Yes No **Why?**

Meal/Snack location:

Dining Table	Restaurant	In front of TV/Computer
In bed	Automobile	Other (Explain)

Beverage Consumed:

Soda	Diet soda/seltzer water	Tap/bottled water
Milk/dairy alternative	Other (Explain)	

Reason for Eating:

Nourishment	Health	Social Activity/Group Gathering
Coping with feelings	Controlling Emotions	Other (Explain)

Reason for Exercise: (Check or circle the major reasons)

Appearance/Weight Maintenance	Fitness/Health Management
Stress/Emotions/Mood or Feeling Management	Socializing

At the beginning, during, or conclusion of the meal/snack/exercise, I felt: (Circle all that apply to any phase of this session)

Bad	Numb	Panic	Empowered	Distressed	Successful
Worried	Anxious	Sad	Depressed	Relief	Motivated
Fear	Lonely	Angry	Contempt	Calm	Self-Disciplined
Comfort	Misery	Control	Driven	Soothed	Traumatized
Shame	Guilt	Tired	Hungry	Other (List)	

ACTIVITY REFLECTION

Journal some thoughts about the meal or snack you selected or the exercise you undertook. Why did you select what you did? How did the choices relate to the rules, habits, and rituals your internal critic helped you set up?

EMOTION REFLECTION

Journal about how the activity reflected the emotions you identified that went along with the activity. What brought the feelings/emotions on? Did they change during the session? What helped them change? Why did you select food/exercise as an outlet for those feelings?

When you complete your last session of Day 10, move on to the Phase One Reflection.

Phase One Session Log Sheet

Day 1 - Day 10

Complete the log for this food/exercise session. Place a checkmark next to or circle all that apply.

Date: **Day of Week:**   **Time:**   AM/PM

Reason for the session: Meal   Snack   Exercise   Other (Explain)

Who joined you: **Or Circle:**   Ate Alone/Exercised Alone

Did you count calories eaten or expended?   Yes   No   **Why?**

Meal/Snack location:

   Dining Table   Restaurant   In front of TV/Computer
   In bed   Automobile   Other (Explain)

Beverage Consumed:

   Soda   Diet soda/seltzer water   Tap/bottled water
   Milk/dairy alternative   Other (Explain)

Reason for Eating:

   Nourishment   Health   Social Activity/Group Gathering
   Coping with feelings   Controlling Emotions   Other (Explain)

Reason for Exercise: (Check or circle the major reasons)

   Appearance/Weight Maintenance   Fitness/Health Management
   Stress/Emotions/Mood or Feeling Management   Socializing

At the beginning, during, or conclusion of the meal/snack/exercise, I felt: (Circle all that apply to any phase of this session)

Bad	Numb	Panic	Empowered	Distressed	Successful
Worried	Anxious	Sad	Depressed	Relief	Motivated
Fear	Lonely	Angry	Contempt	Calm	Self-Disciplined
Comfort	Misery	Control	Driven	Soothed	Traumatized
Shame	Guilt	Tired	Hungry	Other (List)	

ACTIVITY REFLECTION

Journal some thoughts about the meal or snack you selected or the exercise you undertook. Why did you select what you did? How did the choices relate to the rules, habits, and rituals your internal critic helped you set up?

EMOTION REFLECTION

Journal about how the activity reflected the emotions you identified that went along with the activity. What brought the feelings/emotions on? Did they change during the session? What helped them change? Why did you select food/exercise as an outlet for those feelings?

When you complete your last session of Day 10, move on to the Phase One Reflection.

Phase One Session Log Sheet

Day 1 - Day 10

Complete the log for this food/exercise session. Place a checkmark next to or circle all that apply.

Date: **Day of Week:** **Time:** AM/PM

Reason for the session: Meal Snack Exercise Other (Explain)

Who joined you: **Or Circle:** Ate Alone/Exercised Alone

Did you count calories eaten or expended? Yes No **Why?**

Meal/Snack location:

Dining Table	Restaurant	In front of TV/Computer
In bed	Automobile	Other (Explain)

Beverage Consumed:

Soda	Diet soda/seltzer water	Tap/bottled water
Milk/dairy alternative	Other (Explain)	

Reason for Eating:

Nourishment	Health	Social Activity/Group Gathering
Coping with feelings	Controlling Emotions	Other (Explain)

Reason for Exercise: (Check or circle the major reasons)

Appearance/Weight Maintenance	Fitness/Health Management
Stress/Emotions/Mood or Feeling Management	Socializing

At the beginning, during, or conclusion of the meal/snack/exercise, I felt: (Circle all that apply to any phase of this session)

Bad	Numb	Panic	Empowered	Distressed	Successful
Worried	Anxious	Sad	Depressed	Relief	Motivated
Fear	Lonely	Angry	Contempt	Calm	Self-Disciplined
Comfort	Misery	Control	Driven	Soothed	Traumatized
Shame	Guilt	Tired	Hungry	Other (List)	

ACTIVITY REFLECTION

Journal some thoughts about the meal or snack you selected or the exercise you undertook. Why did you select what you did? How did the choices relate to the rules, habits, and rituals your internal critic helped you set up?

EMOTION REFLECTION

Journal about how the activity reflected the emotions you identified that went along with the activity. What brought the feelings/emotions on? Did they change during the session? What helped them change? Why did you select food/exercise as an outlet for those feelings?

When you complete your last session of Day 10, move on to the Phase One Reflection.

Phase One Session Log Sheet

Day 1 - Day 10

Complete the log for this food/exercise session. Place a checkmark next to or circle all that apply.

Date: **Day of Week:** **Time:** AM/PM

Reason for the session: Meal Snack Exercise Other (Explain)

Who joined you: **Or Circle:** Ate Alone/Exercised Alone

Did you count calories eaten or expended? Yes No **Why?**

Meal/Snack location:

Dining Table	Restaurant	In front of TV/Computer
In bed	Automobile	Other (Explain)

Beverage Consumed:

Soda	Diet soda/seltzer water	Tap/bottled water
Milk/dairy alternative	Other (Explain)	

Reason for Eating:

Nourishment	Health	Social Activity/Group Gathering
Coping with feelings	Controlling Emotions	Other (Explain)

Reason for Exercise: (Check or circle the major reasons)

Appearance/Weight Maintenance	Fitness/Health Management
Stress/Emotions/Mood or Feeling Management	Socializing

At the beginning, during, or conclusion of the meal/snack/exercise, I felt: (Circle all that apply to any phase of this session)

Bad	Numb	Panic	Empowered	Distressed	Successful
Worried	Anxious	Sad	Depressed	Relief	Motivated
Fear	Lonely	Angry	Contempt	Calm	Self-Disciplined
Comfort	Misery	Control	Driven	Soothed	Traumatized
Shame	Guilt	Tired	Hungry	Other (List)	

ACTIVITY REFLECTION

Journal some thoughts about the meal or snack you selected or the exercise you undertook. Why did you select what you did? How did the choices relate to the rules, habits, and rituals your internal critic helped you set up?

EMOTION REFLECTION

Journal about how the activity reflected the emotions you identified that went along with the activity. What brought the feelings/emotions on? Did they change during the session? What helped them change? Why did you select food/exercise as an outlet for those feelings?

When you complete your last session of Day 10, move on to the Phase One Reflection.

Phase One Session Log Sheet

Day 1 - Day 10

Complete the log for this food/exercise session. Place a checkmark next to or circle all that apply.

Date: **Day of Week:** **Time:** AM/PM

Reason for the session: Meal Snack Exercise Other (Explain)

Who joined you: **Or Circle:** Ate Alone/Exercised Alone

Did you count calories eaten or expended? Yes No **Why?**

Meal/Snack location:

   Dining Table Restaurant In front of TV/Computer
   In bed Automobile Other (Explain)

Beverage Consumed:

   Soda Diet soda/seltzer water Tap/bottled water
   Milk/dairy alternative Other (Explain)

Reason for Eating:

   Nourishment Health Social Activity/Group Gathering
   Coping with feelings Controlling Emotions Other (Explain)

Reason for Exercise: (Check or circle the major reasons)

   Appearance/Weight Maintenance Fitness/Health Management
   Stress/Emotions/Mood or Feeling Management Socializing

At the beginning, during, or conclusion of the meal/snack/exercise, I felt: (Circle all that apply to any phase of this session)

Bad	Numb	Panic	Empowered	Distressed	Successful
Worried	Anxious	Sad	Depressed	Relief	Motivated
Fear	Lonely	Angry	Contempt	Calm	Self-Disciplined
Comfort	Misery	Control	Driven	Soothed	Traumatized
Shame	Guilt	Tired	Hungry	Other (List)	

ACTIVITY REFLECTION

Journal some thoughts about the meal or snack you selected or the exercise you undertook. Why did you select what you did? How did the choices relate to the rules, habits, and rituals your internal critic helped you set up?

EMOTION REFLECTION

Journal about how the activity reflected the emotions you identified that went along with the activity. What brought the feelings/emotions on? Did they change during the session? What helped them change? Why did you select food/exercise as an outlet for those feelings?

When you complete your last session of Day 10, move on to the Phase One Reflection.

Phase One Session Log Sheet

Day 1 - Day 10

Complete the log for this food/exercise session. Place a checkmark next to or circle all that apply.

Date: **Day of Week:**   **Time:**   AM/PM

Reason for the session: Meal   Snack   Exercise   Other (Explain)

Who joined you: **Or Circle:**   Ate Alone/Exercised Alone

Did you count calories eaten or expended?   Yes   No   **Why?**

Meal/Snack location:

    Dining Table   Restaurant   In front of TV/Computer
    In bed   Automobile   Other (Explain)

Beverage Consumed:

    Soda   Diet soda/seltzer water   Tap/bottled water
    Milk/dairy alternative   Other (Explain)

Reason for Eating:

    Nourishment   Health   Social Activity/Group Gathering
    Coping with feelings   Controlling Emotions   Other (Explain)

Reason for Exercise: (Check or circle the major reasons)

    Appearance/Weight Maintenance   Fitness/Health Management
    Stress/Emotions/Mood or Feeling Management   Socializing

At the beginning, during, or conclusion of the meal/snack/exercise, I felt: (Circle all that apply to any phase of this session)

Bad	Numb	Panic	Empowered	Distressed	Successful
Worried	Anxious	Sad	Depressed	Relief	Motivated
Fear	Lonely	Angry	Contempt	Calm	Self-Disciplined
Comfort	Misery	Control	Driven	Soothed	Traumatized
Shame	Guilt	Tired	Hungry	Other (List)	

Activity Reflection

Journal some thoughts about the meal or snack you selected or the exercise you undertook. Why did you select what you did? How did the choices relate to the rules, habits, and rituals your internal critic helped you set up?

Emotion Reflection

Journal about how the activity reflected the emotions you identified that went along with the activity. What brought the feelings/emotions on? Did they change during the session? What helped them change? Why did you select food/exercise as an outlet for those feelings?

When you complete your last session of Day 10, move on to the Phase One Reflection.

Phase One Session Log Sheet

Day 1 - Day 10

Complete the log for this food/exercise session. Place a checkmark next to or circle all that apply.

Date: **Day of Week:**   **Time:**   AM/PM

Reason for the session: Meal   Snack   Exercise   Other (Explain)

Who joined you: **Or Circle:**   Ate Alone/Exercised Alone

Did you count calories eaten or expended?   Yes   No   **Why?**

Meal/Snack location:

Dining Table	Restaurant	In front of TV/Computer
In bed	Automobile	Other (Explain)

Beverage Consumed:

Soda	Diet soda/seltzer water	Tap/bottled water
Milk/dairy alternative	Other (Explain)	

Reason for Eating:

Nourishment	Health	Social Activity/Group Gathering
Coping with feelings	Controlling Emotions	Other (Explain)

Reason for Exercise: (Check or circle the major reasons)

Appearance/Weight Maintenance	Fitness/Health Management
Stress/Emotions/Mood or Feeling Management	Socializing

At the beginning, during, or conclusion of the meal/snack/exercise, I felt: (Circle all that apply to any phase of this session)

Bad	Numb	Panic	Empowered	Distressed	Successful
Worried	Anxious	Sad	Depressed	Relief	Motivated
Fear	Lonely	Angry	Contempt	Calm	Self-Disciplined
Comfort	Misery	Control	Driven	Soothed	Traumatized
Shame	Guilt	Tired	Hungry	Other (List)	

ACTIVITY REFLECTION

Journal some thoughts about the meal or snack you selected or the exercise you undertook. Why did you select what you did? How did the choices relate to the rules, habits, and rituals your internal critic helped you set up?

EMOTION REFLECTION

Journal about how the activity reflected the emotions you identified that went along with the activity. What brought the feelings/emotions on? Did they change during the session? What helped them change? Why did you select food/exercise as an outlet for those feelings?

When you complete your last session of Day 10, move on to the Phase One Reflection.

Phase One Session Log Sheet

Day 1 - Day 10

Complete the log for this food/exercise session. Place a checkmark next to or circle all that apply.

Date:　　　　　　　　　**Day of Week:**　　　　　　　　**Time:**　　　　　AM/PM

Reason for the session:　　Meal　　　　Snack　　　　Exercise　　　　Other (Explain)

Who joined you:　　　　　　　　　　**Or Circle:**　　　　　Ate Alone/Exercised Alone

Did you count calories eaten or expended?　　Yes　　　No　　**Why?**

Meal/Snack location:

Dining Table	Restaurant	In front of TV/Computer
In bed	Automobile	Other (Explain)

Beverage Consumed:

Soda	Diet soda/seltzer water	Tap/bottled water
Milk/dairy alternative	Other (Explain)	

Reason for Eating:

Nourishment	Health	Social Activity/Group Gathering
Coping with feelings	Controlling Emotions	Other (Explain)

Reason for Exercise: (Check or circle the major reasons)

Appearance/Weight Maintenance	Fitness/Health Management
Stress/Emotions/Mood or Feeling Management	Socializing

At the beginning, during, or conclusion of the meal/snack/exercise, I felt: (Circle all that apply to any phase of this session)

Bad	Numb	Panic	Empowered	Distressed	Successful
Worried	Anxious	Sad	Depressed	Relief	Motivated
Fear	Lonely	Angry	Contempt	Calm	Self-Disciplined
Comfort	Misery	Control	Driven	Soothed	Traumatized
Shame	Guilt	Tired	Hungry	Other (List)	

ACTIVITY REFLECTION

Journal some thoughts about the meal or snack you selected or the exercise you undertook. Why did you select what you did? How did the choices relate to the rules, habits, and rituals your internal critic helped you set up?

EMOTION REFLECTION

Journal about how the activity reflected the emotions you identified that went along with the activity. What brought the feelings/emotions on? Did they change during the session? What helped them change? Why did you select food/exercise as an outlet for those feelings?

When you complete your last session of Day 10, move on to the Phase One Reflection.

Phase One Session Log Sheet

Day 1 - Day 10

Complete the log for this food/exercise session. Place a checkmark next to or circle all that apply.

Date:　　　　　　　　**Day of Week:**　　　　　　　　**Time:**　　　AM/PM

Reason for the session:　　Meal　　　Snack　　　Exercise　　　Other (Explain)

Who joined you:　　　　　　　　**Or Circle:**　　　Ate Alone/Exercised Alone

Did you count calories eaten or expended?　Yes　　No　　**Why?**

Meal/Snack location:

Dining Table	Restaurant	In front of TV/Computer
In bed	Automobile	Other (Explain)

Beverage Consumed:

Soda	Diet soda/seltzer water	Tap/bottled water
Milk/dairy alternative	Other (Explain)	

Reason for Eating:

Nourishment	Health	Social Activity/Group Gathering
Coping with feelings	Controlling Emotions	Other (Explain)

Reason for Exercise: (Check or circle the major reasons)

Appearance/Weight Maintenance	Fitness/Health Management
Stress/Emotions/Mood or Feeling Management	Socializing

At the beginning, during, or conclusion of the meal/snack/exercise, I felt: (Circle all that apply to any phase of this session)

Bad	Numb	Panic	Empowered	Distressed	Successful
Worried	Anxious	Sad	Depressed	Relief	Motivated
Fear	Lonely	Angry	Contempt	Calm	Self-Disciplined
Comfort	Misery	Control	Driven	Soothed	Traumatized
Shame	Guilt	Tired	Hungry	Other (List)	

ACTIVITY REFLECTION

Journal some thoughts about the meal or snack you selected or the exercise you undertook. Why did you select what you did? How did the choices relate to the rules, habits, and rituals your internal critic helped you set up?

EMOTION REFLECTION

Journal about how the activity reflected the emotions you identified that went along with the activity. What brought the feelings/emotions on? Did they change during the session? What helped them change? Why did you select food/exercise as an outlet for those feelings?

When you complete your last session of Day 10, move on to the Phase One Reflection.

Phase One Session Log Sheet

Day 1 - Day 10

Complete the log for this food/exercise session. Place a checkmark next to or circle all that apply.

Date: **Day of Week:** **Time:**   AM/PM

Reason for the session: Meal   Snack   Exercise   Other (Explain)

Who joined you: **Or Circle:**   Ate Alone/Exercised Alone

Did you count calories eaten or expended?   Yes   No   **Why?**

Meal/Snack location:

Dining Table	Restaurant	In front of TV/Computer
In bed	Automobile	Other (Explain)

Beverage Consumed:

Soda	Diet soda/seltzer water	Tap/bottled water
Milk/dairy alternative	Other (Explain)	

Reason for Eating:

Nourishment	Health	Social Activity/Group Gathering
Coping with feelings	Controlling Emotions	Other (Explain)

Reason for Exercise: (Check or circle the major reasons)

Appearance/Weight Maintenance	Fitness/Health Management
Stress/Emotions/Mood or Feeling Management	Socializing

At the beginning, during, or conclusion of the meal/snack/exercise, I felt: (Circle all that apply to any phase of this session)

Bad	Numb	Panic	Empowered	Distressed	Successful
Worried	Anxious	Sad	Depressed	Relief	Motivated
Fear	Lonely	Angry	Contempt	Calm	Self-Disciplined
Comfort	Misery	Control	Driven	Soothed	Traumatized
Shame	Guilt	Tired	Hungry	Other (List)	

ACTIVITY REFLECTION

Journal some thoughts about the meal or snack you selected or the exercise you undertook. Why did you select what you did? How did the choices relate to the rules, habits, and rituals your internal critic helped you set up?

EMOTION REFLECTION

Journal about how the activity reflected the emotions you identified that went along with the activity. What brought the feelings/emotions on? Did they change during the session? What helped them change? Why did you select food/exercise as an outlet for those feelings?

When you complete your last session of Day 10, move on to the Phase One Reflection.

Phase One Session Log Sheet

Day 1 - Day 10

Complete the log for this food/exercise session. Place a checkmark next to or circle all that apply.

Date:　　　　　　　　**Day of Week:**　　　　　　　　**Time:**　　　　AM/PM

Reason for the session:　　Meal　　　　Snack　　　　Exercise　　　　Other (Explain)

Who joined you:　　　　　　　　**Or Circle:**　　　　Ate Alone/Exercised Alone

Did you count calories eaten or expended?　　Yes　　　No　　**Why?**

Meal/Snack location:

　　Dining Table　　　　　　Restaurant　　　　　　　　　In front of TV/Computer
　　In bed　　　　　　　　　Automobile　　　　　　　　　Other (Explain)

Beverage Consumed:

　　Soda　　　　　　　　　　Diet soda/seltzer water　　　Tap/bottled water
　　Milk/dairy alternative　　Other (Explain)

Reason for Eating:

　　Nourishment　　　　　　Health　　　　　　　　　　　Social Activity/Group Gathering
　　Coping with feelings　　Controlling Emotions　　　　Other (Explain)

Reason for Exercise: (Check or circle the major reasons)

　　Appearance/Weight Maintenance　　　　　　　　　　Fitness/Health Management
　　Stress/Emotions/Mood or Feeling Management　　　Socializing

At the beginning, during, or conclusion of the meal/snack/exercise, I felt: (Circle all that apply to any phase of this session)

Bad	Numb	Panic	Empowered	Distressed	Successful
Worried	Anxious	Sad	Depressed	Relief	Motivated
Fear	Lonely	Angry	Contempt	Calm	Self-Disciplined
Comfort	Misery	Control	Driven	Soothed	Traumatized
Shame	Guilt	Tired	Hungry	Other (List)	

ACTIVITY REFLECTION

Journal some thoughts about the meal or snack you selected or the exercise you undertook. Why did you select what you did? How did the choices relate to the rules, habits, and rituals your internal critic helped you set up?

EMOTION REFLECTION

Journal about how the activity reflected the emotions you identified that went along with the activity. What brought the feelings/emotions on? Did they change during the session? What helped them change? Why did you select food/exercise as an outlet for those feelings?

When you complete your last session of Day 10, move on to the Phase One Reflection.

Phase One Session Log Sheet

Day 1 - Day 10

Complete the log for this food/exercise session. Place a checkmark next to or circle all that apply.

Date: **Day of Week:**   **Time:**   AM/PM

Reason for the session: Meal   Snack   Exercise   Other (Explain)

Who joined you: **Or Circle:**   Ate Alone/Exercised Alone

Did you count calories eaten or expended?   Yes   No   **Why?**

Meal/Snack location:

   Dining Table   Restaurant   In front of TV/Computer
   In bed   Automobile   Other (Explain)

Beverage Consumed:

   Soda   Diet soda/seltzer water   Tap/bottled water
   Milk/dairy alternative   Other (Explain)

Reason for Eating:

   Nourishment   Health   Social Activity/Group Gathering
   Coping with feelings   Controlling Emotions   Other (Explain)

Reason for Exercise: (Check or circle the major reasons)

   Appearance/Weight Maintenance   Fitness/Health Management
   Stress/Emotions/Mood or Feeling Management   Socializing

At the beginning, during, or conclusion of the meal/snack/exercise, I felt: (Circle all that apply to any phase of this session)

Bad	Numb	Panic	Empowered	Distressed	Successful
Worried	Anxious	Sad	Depressed	Relief	Motivated
Fear	Lonely	Angry	Contempt	Calm	Self-Disciplined
Comfort	Misery	Control	Driven	Soothed	Traumatized
Shame	Guilt	Tired	Hungry	Other (List)	

ACTIVITY REFLECTION

Journal some thoughts about the meal or snack you selected or the exercise you undertook. Why did you select what you did? How did the choices relate to the rules, habits, and rituals your internal critic helped you set up?

EMOTION REFLECTION

Journal about how the activity reflected the emotions you identified that went along with the activity. What brought the feelings/emotions on? Did they change during the session? What helped them change? Why did you select food/exercise as an outlet for those feelings?

When you complete your last session of Day 10, move on to the Phase One Reflection.

Phase One Session Log Sheet

Day 1 - Day 10

Complete the log for this food/exercise session. Place a checkmark next to or circle all that apply.

Date: **Day of Week:** **Time:** AM/PM

Reason for the session: Meal Snack Exercise Other (Explain)

Who joined you: **Or Circle:** Ate Alone/Exercised Alone

Did you count calories eaten or expended? Yes No **Why?**

Meal/Snack location:

   Dining Table Restaurant In front of TV/Computer
   In bed Automobile Other (Explain)

Beverage Consumed:

   Soda Diet soda/seltzer water Tap/bottled water
   Milk/dairy alternative Other (Explain)

Reason for Eating:

   Nourishment Health Social Activity/Group Gathering
   Coping with feelings Controlling Emotions Other (Explain)

Reason for Exercise: (Check or circle the major reasons)

   Appearance/Weight Maintenance Fitness/Health Management
   Stress/Emotions/Mood or Feeling Management Socializing

At the beginning, during, or conclusion of the meal/snack/exercise, I felt: (Circle all that apply to any phase of this session)

Bad	Numb	Panic	Empowered	Distressed	Successful
Worried	Anxious	Sad	Depressed	Relief	Motivated
Fear	Lonely	Angry	Contempt	Calm	Self-Disciplined
Comfort	Misery	Control	Driven	Soothed	Traumatized
Shame	Guilt	Tired	Hungry	Other (List)	

Activity Reflection

Journal some thoughts about the meal or snack you selected or the exercise you undertook. Why did you select what you did? How did the choices relate to the rules, habits, and rituals your internal critic helped you set up?

Emotion Reflection

Journal about how the activity reflected the emotions you identified that went along with the activity. What brought the feelings/emotions on? Did they change during the session? What helped them change? Why did you select food/exercise as an outlet for those feelings?

When you complete your last session of Day 10, move on to the Phase One Reflection.

Phase One Session Log Sheet

Day 1 - Day 10

Complete the log for this food/exercise session. Place a checkmark next to or circle all that apply.

Date: **Day of Week:**   **Time:**   AM/PM

Reason for the session: Meal   Snack   Exercise   Other (Explain)

Who joined you: **Or Circle:**   Ate Alone/Exercised Alone

Did you count calories eaten or expended?   Yes   No   **Why?**

Meal/Snack location:

Dining Table	Restaurant	In front of TV/Computer
In bed	Automobile	Other (Explain)

Beverage Consumed:

Soda	Diet soda/seltzer water	Tap/bottled water
Milk/dairy alternative	Other (Explain)	

Reason for Eating:

Nourishment	Health	Social Activity/Group Gathering
Coping with feelings	Controlling Emotions	Other (Explain)

Reason for Exercise: (Check or circle the major reasons)

Appearance/Weight Maintenance	Fitness/Health Management
Stress/Emotions/Mood or Feeling Management	Socializing

At the beginning, during, or conclusion of the meal/snack/exercise, I felt: (Circle all that apply to any phase of this session)

Bad	Numb	Panic	Empowered	Distressed	Successful
Worried	Anxious	Sad	Depressed	Relief	Motivated
Fear	Lonely	Angry	Contempt	Calm	Self-Disciplined
Comfort	Misery	Control	Driven	Soothed	Traumatized
Shame	Guilt	Tired	Hungry	Other (List)	

ACTIVITY REFLECTION

Journal some thoughts about the meal or snack you selected or the exercise you undertook. Why did you select what you did? How did the choices relate to the rules, habits, and rituals your internal critic helped you set up?

EMOTION REFLECTION

Journal about how the activity reflected the emotions you identified that went along with the activity. What brought the feelings/emotions on? Did they change during the session? What helped them change? Why did you select food/exercise as an outlet for those feelings?

When you complete your last session of Day 10, move on to the Phase One Reflection.

Phase One Session Log Sheet

Day 1 - Day 10

Complete the log for this food/exercise session. Place a checkmark next to or circle all that apply.

Date:　　　　　　　　**Day of Week:**　　　　　　　**Time:**　　　　AM/PM

Reason for the session:　　Meal　　　Snack　　　Exercise　　　Other (Explain)

Who joined you:　　　　　　　　**Or Circle:**　　　　Ate Alone/Exercised Alone

Did you count calories eaten or expended?　　Yes　　No　　**Why?**

Meal/Snack location:

Dining Table	Restaurant	In front of TV/Computer
In bed	Automobile	Other (Explain)

Beverage Consumed:

Soda	Diet soda/seltzer water	Tap/bottled water
Milk/dairy alternative	Other (Explain)	

Reason for Eating:

Nourishment	Health	Social Activity/Group Gathering
Coping with feelings	Controlling Emotions	Other (Explain)

Reason for Exercise: (Check or circle the major reasons)

Appearance/Weight Maintenance	Fitness/Health Management
Stress/Emotions/Mood or Feeling Management	Socializing

At the beginning, during, or conclusion of the meal/snack/exercise, I felt: (Circle all that apply to any phase of this session)

Bad	Numb	Panic	Empowered	Distressed	Successful
Worried	Anxious	Sad	Depressed	Relief	Motivated
Fear	Lonely	Angry	Contempt	Calm	Self-Disciplined
Comfort	Misery	Control	Driven	Soothed	Traumatized
Shame	Guilt	Tired	Hungry	Other (List)	

ACTIVITY REFLECTION

Journal some thoughts about the meal or snack you selected or the exercise you undertook. Why did you select what you did? How did the choices relate to the rules, habits, and rituals your internal critic helped you set up?

EMOTION REFLECTION

Journal about how the activity reflected the emotions you identified that went along with the activity. What brought the feelings/emotions on? Did they change during the session? What helped them change? Why did you select food/exercise as an outlet for those feelings?

When you complete your last session of Day 10, move on to the Phase One Reflection.

Phase One Session Log Sheet

Day 1 - Day 10

Complete the log for this food/exercise session. Place a checkmark next to or circle all that apply.

Date: **Day of Week:**   **Time:**   AM/PM

Reason for the session: Meal   Snack   Exercise   Other (Explain)

Who joined you: **Or Circle:**   Ate Alone/Exercised Alone

Did you count calories eaten or expended?   Yes   No   **Why?**

Meal/Snack location:

Dining Table	Restaurant	In front of TV/Computer
In bed	Automobile	Other (Explain)

Beverage Consumed:

Soda	Diet soda/seltzer water	Tap/bottled water
Milk/dairy alternative	Other (Explain)	

Reason for Eating:

Nourishment	Health	Social Activity/Group Gathering
Coping with feelings	Controlling Emotions	Other (Explain)

Reason for Exercise: (Check or circle the major reasons)

Appearance/Weight Maintenance	Fitness/Health Management
Stress/Emotions/Mood or Feeling Management	Socializing

At the beginning, during, or conclusion of the meal/snack/exercise, I felt: (Circle all that apply to any phase of this session)

Bad	Numb	Panic	Empowered	Distressed	Successful
Worried	Anxious	Sad	Depressed	Relief	Motivated
Fear	Lonely	Angry	Contempt	Calm	Self-Disciplined
Comfort	Misery	Control	Driven	Soothed	Traumatized
Shame	Guilt	Tired	Hungry	Other (List)	

Activity Reflection

Journal some thoughts about the meal or snack you selected or the exercise you undertook. Why did you select what you did? How did the choices relate to the rules, habits, and rituals your internal critic helped you set up?

Emotion Reflection

Journal about how the activity reflected the emotions you identified that went along with the activity. What brought the feelings/emotions on? Did they change during the session? What helped them change? Why did you select food/exercise as an outlet for those feelings?

When you complete your last session of Day 10, move on to the Phase One Reflection.

Phase One Session Log Sheet

Day 1 - Day 10

Complete the log for this food/exercise session. Place a checkmark next to or circle all that apply.

Date: **Day of Week:** **Time:** AM/PM

Reason for the session: Meal Snack Exercise Other (Explain)

Who joined you: **Or Circle:** Ate Alone/Exercised Alone

Did you count calories eaten or expended? Yes No **Why?**

Meal/Snack location:

Dining Table	Restaurant	In front of TV/Computer
In bed	Automobile	Other (Explain)

Beverage Consumed:

Soda	Diet soda/seltzer water	Tap/bottled water
Milk/dairy alternative	Other (Explain)	

Reason for Eating:

Nourishment	Health	Social Activity/Group Gathering
Coping with feelings	Controlling Emotions	Other (Explain)

Reason for Exercise: (Check or circle the major reasons)

Appearance/Weight Maintenance	Fitness/Health Management
Stress/Emotions/Mood or Feeling Management	Socializing

At the beginning, during, or conclusion of the meal/snack/exercise, I felt: (Circle all that apply to any phase of this session)

Bad	Numb	Panic	Empowered	Distressed	Successful
Worried	Anxious	Sad	Depressed	Relief	Motivated
Fear	Lonely	Angry	Contempt	Calm	Self-Disciplined
Comfort	Misery	Control	Driven	Soothed	Traumatized
Shame	Guilt	Tired	Hungry	Other (List)	

ACTIVITY REFLECTION

Journal some thoughts about the meal or snack you selected or the exercise you undertook. Why did you select what you did? How did the choices relate to the rules, habits, and rituals your internal critic helped you set up?

EMOTION REFLECTION

Journal about how the activity reflected the emotions you identified that went along with the activity. What brought the feelings/emotions on? Did they change during the session? What helped them change? Why did you select food/exercise as an outlet for those feelings?

When you complete your last session of Day 10, move on to the Phase One Reflection.

Phase One Session Log Sheet

Day 1 - Day 10

Complete the log for this food/exercise session. Place a checkmark next to or circle all that apply.

Date: **Day of Week:**   **Time:**   AM/PM

Reason for the session: Meal   Snack   Exercise   Other (Explain)

Who joined you: **Or Circle:**   Ate Alone/Exercised Alone

Did you count calories eaten or expended?   Yes   No   **Why?**

Meal/Snack location:

Dining Table	Restaurant	In front of TV/Computer
In bed	Automobile	Other (Explain)

Beverage Consumed:

Soda	Diet soda/seltzer water	Tap/bottled water
Milk/dairy alternative	Other (Explain)	

Reason for Eating:

Nourishment	Health	Social Activity/Group Gathering
Coping with feelings	Controlling Emotions	Other (Explain)

Reason for Exercise: (Check or circle the major reasons)

Appearance/Weight Maintenance	Fitness/Health Management
Stress/Emotions/Mood or Feeling Management	Socializing

At the beginning, during, or conclusion of the meal/snack/exercise, I felt: (Circle all that apply to any phase of this session)

Bad	Numb	Panic	Empowered	Distressed	Successful
Worried	Anxious	Sad	Depressed	Relief	Motivated
Fear	Lonely	Angry	Contempt	Calm	Self-Disciplined
Comfort	Misery	Control	Driven	Soothed	Traumatized
Shame	Guilt	Tired	Hungry	Other (List)	

ACTIVITY REFLECTION

Journal some thoughts about the meal or snack you selected or the exercise you undertook. Why did you select what you did? How did the choices relate to the rules, habits, and rituals your internal critic helped you set up?

EMOTION REFLECTION

Journal about how the activity reflected the emotions you identified that went along with the activity. What brought the feelings/emotions on? Did they change during the session? What helped them change? Why did you select food/exercise as an outlet for those feelings?

When you complete your last session of Day 10, move on to the Phase One Reflection.

Phase One Session Log Sheet

Day 1 - Day 10

Complete the log for this food/exercise session. Place a checkmark next to or circle all that apply.

Date: **Day of Week:** **Time:** AM/PM

Reason for the session: Meal Snack Exercise Other (Explain)

Who joined you: **Or Circle:** Ate Alone/Exercised Alone

Did you count calories eaten or expended? Yes No **Why?**

Meal/Snack location:

Dining Table	Restaurant	In front of TV/Computer
In bed	Automobile	Other (Explain)

Beverage Consumed:

Soda	Diet soda/seltzer water	Tap/bottled water
Milk/dairy alternative	Other (Explain)	

Reason for Eating:

Nourishment	Health	Social Activity/Group Gathering
Coping with feelings	Controlling Emotions	Other (Explain)

Reason for Exercise: (Check or circle the major reasons)

Appearance/Weight Maintenance	Fitness/Health Management
Stress/Emotions/Mood or Feeling Management	Socializing

At the beginning, during, or conclusion of the meal/snack/exercise, I felt: (Circle all that apply to any phase of this session)

Bad	Numb	Panic	Empowered	Distressed	Successful
Worried	Anxious	Sad	Depressed	Relief	Motivated
Fear	Lonely	Angry	Contempt	Calm	Self-Disciplined
Comfort	Misery	Control	Driven	Soothed	Traumatized
Shame	Guilt	Tired	Hungry	Other (List)	

Activity Reflection

Journal some thoughts about the meal or snack you selected or the exercise you undertook. Why did you select what you did? How did the choices relate to the rules, habits, and rituals your internal critic helped you set up?

Emotion Reflection

Journal about how the activity reflected the emotions you identified that went along with the activity. What brought the feelings/emotions on? Did they change during the session? What helped them change? Why did you select food/exercise as an outlet for those feelings?

When you complete your last session of Day 10, move on to the Phase One Reflection.

Phase One Session Log Sheet

Day 1 - Day 10

Complete the log for this food/exercise session. Place a checkmark next to or circle all that apply.

Date: **Day of Week:**   **Time:**   AM/PM

Reason for the session: Meal   Snack   Exercise   Other (Explain)

Who joined you: **Or Circle:**   Ate Alone/Exercised Alone

Did you count calories eaten or expended?   Yes   No   **Why?**

Meal/Snack location:

Dining Table	Restaurant	In front of TV/Computer
In bed	Automobile	Other (Explain)

Beverage Consumed:

Soda	Diet soda/seltzer water	Tap/bottled water
Milk/dairy alternative	Other (Explain)	

Reason for Eating:

Nourishment	Health	Social Activity/Group Gathering
Coping with feelings	Controlling Emotions	Other (Explain)

Reason for Exercise: (Check or circle the major reasons)

Appearance/Weight Maintenance	Fitness/Health Management
Stress/Emotions/Mood or Feeling Management	Socializing

At the beginning, during, or conclusion of the meal/snack/exercise, I felt: (Circle all that apply to any phase of this session)

Bad	Numb	Panic	Empowered	Distressed	Successful
Worried	Anxious	Sad	Depressed	Relief	Motivated
Fear	Lonely	Angry	Contempt	Calm	Self-Disciplined
Comfort	Misery	Control	Driven	Soothed	Traumatized
Shame	Guilt	Tired	Hungry	Other (List)	

Activity Reflection

Journal some thoughts about the meal or snack you selected or the exercise you undertook. Why did you select what you did? How did the choices relate to the rules, habits, and rituals your internal critic helped you set up?

Emotion Reflection

Journal about how the activity reflected the emotions you identified that went along with the activity. What brought the feelings/emotions on? Did they change during the session? What helped them change? Why did you select food/exercise as an outlet for those feelings?

When you complete your last session of Day 10, move on to the Phase One Reflection.

Phase One Session Log Sheet

Day 1 - Day 10

Complete the log for this food/exercise session. Place a checkmark next to or circle all that apply.

Date:　　　　　　　　　　**Day of Week:**　　　　　　　　**Time:**　　　　AM/PM

Reason for the session:　　Meal　　　　Snack　　　　Exercise　　　　Other (Explain)

Who joined you:　　　　　　　　**Or Circle:**　　　　Ate Alone/Exercised Alone

Did you count calories eaten or expended?　　Yes　　　No　　**Why?**

Meal/Snack location:

Dining Table	Restaurant	In front of TV/Computer
In bed	Automobile	Other (Explain)

Beverage Consumed:

Soda	Diet soda/seltzer water	Tap/bottled water
Milk/dairy alternative	Other (Explain)	

Reason for Eating:

Nourishment	Health	Social Activity/Group Gathering
Coping with feelings	Controlling Emotions	Other (Explain)

Reason for Exercise: (Check or circle the major reasons)

Appearance/Weight Maintenance	Fitness/Health Management
Stress/Emotions/Mood or Feeling Management	Socializing

At the beginning, during, or conclusion of the meal/snack/exercise, I felt: (Circle all that apply to any phase of this session)

Bad	Numb	Panic	Empowered	Distressed	Successful
Worried	Anxious	Sad	Depressed	Relief	Motivated
Fear	Lonely	Angry	Contempt	Calm	Self-Disciplined
Comfort	Misery	Control	Driven	Soothed	Traumatized
Shame	Guilt	Tired	Hungry	Other (List)	

ACTIVITY REFLECTION

Journal some thoughts about the meal or snack you selected or the exercise you undertook. Why did you select what you did? How did the choices relate to the rules, habits, and rituals your internal critic helped you set up?

EMOTION REFLECTION

Journal about how the activity reflected the emotions you identified that went along with the activity. What brought the feelings/emotions on? Did they change during the session? What helped them change? Why did you select food/exercise as an outlet for those feelings?

When you complete your last session of Day 10, move on to the Phase One Reflection.

Phase One Session Log Sheet

Day 1 - Day 10

Complete the log for this food/exercise session. Place a checkmark next to or circle all that apply.

Date: **Day of Week:** **Time:** AM/PM

Reason for the session: Meal   Snack   Exercise   Other (Explain)

Who joined you: **Or Circle:**   Ate Alone/Exercised Alone

Did you count calories eaten or expended?   Yes   No   **Why?**

Meal/Snack location:

Dining Table	Restaurant	In front of TV/Computer
In bed	Automobile	Other (Explain)

Beverage Consumed:

Soda	Diet soda/seltzer water	Tap/bottled water
Milk/dairy alternative	Other (Explain)	

Reason for Eating:

Nourishment	Health	Social Activity/Group Gathering
Coping with feelings	Controlling Emotions	Other (Explain)

Reason for Exercise: (Check or circle the major reasons)

Appearance/Weight Maintenance	Fitness/Health Management
Stress/Emotions/Mood or Feeling Management	Socializing

At the beginning, during, or conclusion of the meal/snack/exercise, I felt: (Circle all that apply to any phase of this session)

Bad	Numb	Panic	Empowered	Distressed	Successful
Worried	Anxious	Sad	Depressed	Relief	Motivated
Fear	Lonely	Angry	Contempt	Calm	Self-Disciplined
Comfort	Misery	Control	Driven	Soothed	Traumatized
Shame	Guilt	Tired	Hungry	Other (List)	

ACTIVITY REFLECTION

Journal some thoughts about the meal or snack you selected or the exercise you undertook. Why did you select what you did? How did the choices relate to the rules, habits, and rituals your internal critic helped you set up?

EMOTION REFLECTION

Journal about how the activity reflected the emotions you identified that went along with the activity. What brought the feelings/emotions on? Did they change during the session? What helped them change? Why did you select food/exercise as an outlet for those feelings?

When you complete your last session of Day 10, move on to the Phase One Reflection.

Phase One Session Log Sheet

Day 1 - Day 10

Complete the log for this food/exercise session. Place a checkmark next to or circle all that apply.

Date: **Day of Week:**   **Time:**   AM/PM

Reason for the session: Meal   Snack   Exercise   Other (Explain)

Who joined you: **Or Circle:**   Ate Alone/Exercised Alone

Did you count calories eaten or expended?   Yes   No   **Why?**

Meal/Snack location:

    Dining Table   Restaurant   In front of TV/Computer
    In bed   Automobile   Other (Explain)

Beverage Consumed:

    Soda   Diet soda/seltzer water   Tap/bottled water
    Milk/dairy alternative   Other (Explain)

Reason for Eating:

    Nourishment   Health   Social Activity/Group Gathering
    Coping with feelings   Controlling Emotions   Other (Explain)

Reason for Exercise: (Check or circle the major reasons)

    Appearance/Weight Maintenance   Fitness/Health Management
    Stress/Emotions/Mood or Feeling Management   Socializing

At the beginning, during, or conclusion of the meal/snack/exercise, I felt: (Circle all that apply to any phase of this session)

Bad	Numb	Panic	Empowered	Distressed	Successful
Worried	Anxious	Sad	Depressed	Relief	Motivated
Fear	Lonely	Angry	Contempt	Calm	Self-Disciplined
Comfort	Misery	Control	Driven	Soothed	Traumatized
Shame	Guilt	Tired	Hungry	Other (List)	

Activity Reflection

Journal some thoughts about the meal or snack you selected or the exercise you undertook. Why did you select what you did? How did the choices relate to the rules, habits, and rituals your internal critic helped you set up?

Emotion Reflection

Journal about how the activity reflected the emotions you identified that went along with the activity. What brought the feelings/emotions on? Did they change during the session? What helped them change? Why did you select food/exercise as an outlet for those feelings?

When you complete your last session of Day 10, move on to the Phase One Reflection.

Phase One Session Log Sheet

Day 1 - Day 10

Complete the log for this food/exercise session. Place a checkmark next to or circle all that apply.

Date:　　　　　　　　　**Day of Week:**　　　　　　　　**Time:**　　　　AM/PM

Reason for the session:　　Meal　　　　Snack　　　　Exercise　　　　Other (Explain)

Who joined you:　　　　　　　　**Or Circle:**　　　　Ate Alone/Exercised Alone

Did you count calories eaten or expended?　　Yes　　No　　**Why?**

Meal/Snack location:

Dining Table	Restaurant	In front of TV/Computer
In bed	Automobile	Other (Explain)

Beverage Consumed:

Soda	Diet soda/seltzer water	Tap/bottled water
Milk/dairy alternative	Other (Explain)	

Reason for Eating:

Nourishment	Health	Social Activity/Group Gathering
Coping with feelings	Controlling Emotions	Other (Explain)

Reason for Exercise: (Check or circle the major reasons)

Appearance/Weight Maintenance	Fitness/Health Management
Stress/Emotions/Mood or Feeling Management	Socializing

At the beginning, during, or conclusion of the meal/snack/exercise, I felt: (Circle all that apply to any phase of this session)

Bad	Numb	Panic	Empowered	Distressed	Successful
Worried	Anxious	Sad	Depressed	Relief	Motivated
Fear	Lonely	Angry	Contempt	Calm	Self-Disciplined
Comfort	Misery	Control	Driven	Soothed	Traumatized
Shame	Guilt	Tired	Hungry	Other (List)	

ACTIVITY REFLECTION

Journal some thoughts about the meal or snack you selected or the exercise you undertook. Why did you select what you did? How did the choices relate to the rules, habits, and rituals your internal critic helped you set up?

EMOTION REFLECTION

Journal about how the activity reflected the emotions you identified that went along with the activity. What brought the feelings/emotions on? Did they change during the session? What helped them change? Why did you select food/exercise as an outlet for those feelings?

When you complete your last session of Day 10, move on to the Phase One Reflection.

Phase One Session Log Sheet

Day 1 - Day 10

Complete the log for this food/exercise session. Place a checkmark next to or circle all that apply.

Date: **Day of Week:**   **Time:**   AM/PM

Reason for the session: Meal   Snack   Exercise   Other (Explain)

Who joined you: **Or Circle:**   Ate Alone/Exercised Alone

Did you count calories eaten or expended?   Yes   No   **Why?**

Meal/Snack location:

Dining Table	Restaurant	In front of TV/Computer
In bed	Automobile	Other (Explain)

Beverage Consumed:

Soda	Diet soda/seltzer water	Tap/bottled water
Milk/dairy alternative	Other (Explain)	

Reason for Eating:

Nourishment	Health	Social Activity/Group Gathering
Coping with feelings	Controlling Emotions	Other (Explain)

Reason for Exercise: (Check or circle the major reasons)

Appearance/Weight Maintenance	Fitness/Health Management
Stress/Emotions/Mood or Feeling Management	Socializing

At the beginning, during, or conclusion of the meal/snack/exercise, I felt: (Circle all that apply to any phase of this session)

Bad	Numb	Panic	Empowered	Distressed	Successful
Worried	Anxious	Sad	Depressed	Relief	Motivated
Fear	Lonely	Angry	Contempt	Calm	Self-Disciplined
Comfort	Misery	Control	Driven	Soothed	Traumatized
Shame	Guilt	Tired	Hungry	Other (List)	

ACTIVITY REFLECTION

Journal some thoughts about the meal or snack you selected or the exercise you undertook. Why did you select what you did? How did the choices relate to the rules, habits, and rituals your internal critic helped you set up?

EMOTION REFLECTION

Journal about how the activity reflected the emotions you identified that went along with the activity. What brought the feelings/emotions on? Did they change during the session? What helped them change? Why did you select food/exercise as an outlet for those feelings?

When you complete your last session of Day 10, move on to the Phase One Reflection.

Phase One Session Log Sheet

Day 1 - Day 10

Complete the log for this food/exercise session. Place a checkmark next to or circle all that apply.

Date: **Day of Week:** **Time:** AM/PM

Reason for the session: Meal Snack Exercise Other (Explain)

Who joined you: **Or Circle:** Ate Alone/Exercised Alone

Did you count calories eaten or expended? Yes No **Why?**

Meal/Snack location:

Dining Table	Restaurant	In front of TV/Computer
In bed	Automobile	Other (Explain)

Beverage Consumed:

Soda	Diet soda/seltzer water	Tap/bottled water
Milk/dairy alternative	Other (Explain)	

Reason for Eating:

Nourishment	Health	Social Activity/Group Gathering
Coping with feelings	Controlling Emotions	Other (Explain)

Reason for Exercise: (Check or circle the major reasons)

Appearance/Weight Maintenance	Fitness/Health Management
Stress/Emotions/Mood or Feeling Management	Socializing

At the beginning, during, or conclusion of the meal/snack/exercise, I felt: (Circle all that apply to any phase of this session)

Bad	Numb	Panic	Empowered	Distressed	Successful
Worried	Anxious	Sad	Depressed	Relief	Motivated
Fear	Lonely	Angry	Contempt	Calm	Self-Disciplined
Comfort	Misery	Control	Driven	Soothed	Traumatized
Shame	Guilt	Tired	Hungry	Other (List)	

ACTIVITY REFLECTION

Journal some thoughts about the meal or snack you selected or the exercise you undertook. Why did you select what you did? How did the choices relate to the rules, habits, and rituals your internal critic helped you set up?

EMOTION REFLECTION

Journal about how the activity reflected the emotions you identified that went along with the activity. What brought the feelings/emotions on? Did they change during the session? What helped them change? Why did you select food/exercise as an outlet for those feelings?

When you complete your last session of Day 10, move on to the Phase One Reflection.

Phase One Session Log Sheet

Day 1 - Day 10

Complete the log for this food/exercise session. Place a checkmark next to or circle all that apply.

Date: **Day of Week:**   **Time:**   AM/PM

Reason for the session: Meal   Snack   Exercise   Other (Explain)

Who joined you: **Or Circle:**   Ate Alone/Exercised Alone

Did you count calories eaten or expended?   Yes   No   **Why?**

Meal/Snack location:

- Dining Table
- In bed
- Restaurant
- Automobile
- In front of TV/Computer
- Other (Explain)

Beverage Consumed:

- Soda
- Milk/dairy alternative
- Diet soda/seltzer water
- Other (Explain)
- Tap/bottled water

Reason for Eating:

- Nourishment
- Coping with feelings
- Health
- Controlling Emotions
- Social Activity/Group Gathering
- Other (Explain)

Reason for Exercise: (Check or circle the major reasons)

- Appearance/Weight Maintenance
- Stress/Emotions/Mood or Feeling Management
- Fitness/Health Management
- Socializing

At the beginning, during, or conclusion of the meal/snack/exercise, I felt: (Circle all that apply to any phase of this session)

Bad	Numb	Panic	Empowered	Distressed	Successful
Worried	Anxious	Sad	Depressed	Relief	Motivated
Fear	Lonely	Angry	Contempt	Calm	Self-Disciplined
Comfort	Misery	Control	Driven	Soothed	Traumatized
Shame	Guilt	Tired	Hungry	Other (List)	

ACTIVITY REFLECTION

Journal some thoughts about the meal or snack you selected or the exercise you undertook. Why did you select what you did? How did the choices relate to the rules, habits, and rituals your internal critic helped you set up?

EMOTION REFLECTION

Journal about how the activity reflected the emotions you identified that went along with the activity. What brought the feelings/emotions on? Did they change during the session? What helped them change? Why did you select food/exercise as an outlet for those feelings?

When you complete your last session of Day 10, move on to the Phase One Reflection.

Phase One Session Log Sheet

Day 1 - Day 10

Complete the log for this food/exercise session. Place a checkmark next to or circle all that apply.

Date: **Day of Week:**   **Time:**   AM/PM

Reason for the session: Meal   Snack   Exercise   Other (Explain)

Who joined you: **Or Circle:**   Ate Alone/Exercised Alone

Did you count calories eaten or expended?   Yes   No   **Why?**

Meal/Snack location:

Dining Table	Restaurant	In front of TV/Computer
In bed	Automobile	Other (Explain)

Beverage Consumed:

Soda	Diet soda/seltzer water	Tap/bottled water
Milk/dairy alternative	Other (Explain)	

Reason for Eating:

Nourishment	Health	Social Activity/Group Gathering
Coping with feelings	Controlling Emotions	Other (Explain)

Reason for Exercise: (Check or circle the major reasons)

Appearance/Weight Maintenance	Fitness/Health Management
Stress/Emotions/Mood or Feeling Management	Socializing

At the beginning, during, or conclusion of the meal/snack/exercise, I felt: (Circle all that apply to any phase of this session)

Bad	Numb	Panic	Empowered	Distressed	Successful
Worried	Anxious	Sad	Depressed	Relief	Motivated
Fear	Lonely	Angry	Contempt	Calm	Self-Disciplined
Comfort	Misery	Control	Driven	Soothed	Traumatized
Shame	Guilt	Tired	Hungry	Other (List)	

ACTIVITY REFLECTION

Journal some thoughts about the meal or snack you selected or the exercise you undertook. Why did you select what you did? How did the choices relate to the rules, habits, and rituals your internal critic helped you set up?

EMOTION REFLECTION

Journal about how the activity reflected the emotions you identified that went along with the activity. What brought the feelings/emotions on? Did they change during the session? What helped them change? Why did you select food/exercise as an outlet for those feelings?

When you complete your last session of Day 10, move on to the Phase One Reflection.

Phase One Session Log Sheet

Day 1 - Day 10

Complete the log for this food/exercise session. Place a checkmark next to or circle all that apply.

Date: **Day of Week:** **Time:** AM/PM

Reason for the session: Meal Snack Exercise Other (Explain)

Who joined you: **Or Circle:** Ate Alone/Exercised Alone

Did you count calories eaten or expended? Yes No **Why?**

Meal/Snack location:

Dining Table	Restaurant	In front of TV/Computer
In bed	Automobile	Other (Explain)

Beverage Consumed:

Soda	Diet soda/seltzer water	Tap/bottled water
Milk/dairy alternative	Other (Explain)	

Reason for Eating:

Nourishment	Health	Social Activity/Group Gathering
Coping with feelings	Controlling Emotions	Other (Explain)

Reason for Exercise: (Check or circle the major reasons)

Appearance/Weight Maintenance	Fitness/Health Management
Stress/Emotions/Mood or Feeling Management	Socializing

At the beginning, during, or conclusion of the meal/snack/exercise, I felt: (Circle all that apply to any phase of this session)

Bad	Numb	Panic	Empowered	Distressed	Successful
Worried	Anxious	Sad	Depressed	Relief	Motivated
Fear	Lonely	Angry	Contempt	Calm	Self-Disciplined
Comfort	Misery	Control	Driven	Soothed	Traumatized
Shame	Guilt	Tired	Hungry	Other (List)	

ACTIVITY REFLECTION

Journal some thoughts about the meal or snack you selected or the exercise you undertook. Why did you select what you did? How did the choices relate to the rules, habits, and rituals your internal critic helped you set up?

EMOTION REFLECTION

Journal about how the activity reflected the emotions you identified that went along with the activity. What brought the feelings/emotions on? Did they change during the session? What helped them change? Why did you select food/exercise as an outlet for those feelings?

When you complete your last session of Day 10, move on to the Phase One Reflection.

Phase One Session Log Sheet

Day 1 - Day 10

Complete the log for this food/exercise session. Place a checkmark next to or circle all that apply.

Date: **Day of Week:** **Time:** AM/PM

Reason for the session: Meal   Snack   Exercise   Other (Explain)

Who joined you: **Or Circle:**   Ate Alone/Exercised Alone

Did you count calories eaten or expended?   Yes   No   **Why?**

Meal/Snack location:

Dining Table	Restaurant	In front of TV/Computer
In bed	Automobile	Other (Explain)

Beverage Consumed:

Soda	Diet soda/seltzer water	Tap/bottled water
Milk/dairy alternative	Other (Explain)	

Reason for Eating:

Nourishment	Health	Social Activity/Group Gathering
Coping with feelings	Controlling Emotions	Other (Explain)

Reason for Exercise: (Check or circle the major reasons)

Appearance/Weight Maintenance	Fitness/Health Management
Stress/Emotions/Mood or Feeling Management	Socializing

At the beginning, during, or conclusion of the meal/snack/exercise, I felt: (Circle all that apply to any phase of this session)

Bad	Numb	Panic	Empowered	Distressed	Successful
Worried	Anxious	Sad	Depressed	Relief	Motivated
Fear	Lonely	Angry	Contempt	Calm	Self-Disciplined
Comfort	Misery	Control	Driven	Soothed	Traumatized
Shame	Guilt	Tired	Hungry	Other (List)	

ACTIVITY REFLECTION

Journal some thoughts about the meal or snack you selected or the exercise you undertook. Why did you select what you did? How did the choices relate to the rules, habits, and rituals your internal critic helped you set up?

EMOTION REFLECTION

Journal about how the activity reflected the emotions you identified that went along with the activity. What brought the feelings/emotions on? Did they change during the session? What helped them change? Why did you select food/exercise as an outlet for those feelings?

When you complete your last session of Day 10, move on to the Phase One Reflection.

Phase One Session Log Sheet

Day 1 - Day 10

Complete the log for this food/exercise session. Place a checkmark next to or circle all that apply.

Date: **Day of Week:**   **Time:**   AM/PM

Reason for the session: Meal   Snack   Exercise   Other (Explain)

Who joined you: **Or Circle:**   Ate Alone/Exercised Alone

Did you count calories eaten or expended?   Yes   No   **Why?**

Meal/Snack location:

   Dining Table   Restaurant   In front of TV/Computer
   In bed   Automobile   Other (Explain)

Beverage Consumed:

   Soda   Diet soda/seltzer water   Tap/bottled water
   Milk/dairy alternative Other (Explain)

Reason for Eating:

   Nourishment   Health   Social Activity/Group Gathering
   Coping with feelings   Controlling Emotions   Other (Explain)

Reason for Exercise: (Check or circle the major reasons)

   Appearance/Weight Maintenance   Fitness/Health Management
   Stress/Emotions/Mood or Feeling Management Socializing

At the beginning, during, or conclusion of the meal/snack/exercise, I felt: (Circle all that apply to any phase of this session)

Bad	Numb	Panic	Empowered	Distressed	Successful
Worried	Anxious	Sad	Depressed	Relief	Motivated
Fear	Lonely	Angry	Contempt	Calm	Self-Disciplined
Comfort	Misery	Control	Driven	Soothed	Traumatized
Shame	Guilt	Tired	Hungry	Other (List)	

ACTIVITY REFLECTION

Journal some thoughts about the meal or snack you selected or the exercise you undertook. Why did you select what you did? How did the choices relate to the rules, habits, and rituals your internal critic helped you set up?

EMOTION REFLECTION

Journal about how the activity reflected the emotions you identified that went along with the activity. What brought the feelings/emotions on? Did they change during the session? What helped them change? Why did you select food/exercise as an outlet for those feelings?

When you complete your last session of Day 10, move on to the Phase One Reflection.

Phase One Session Log Sheet

Day 1 - Day 10

Complete the log for this food/exercise session. Place a checkmark next to or circle all that apply.

Date: **Day of Week:** **Time:** AM/PM

Reason for the session: Meal Snack Exercise Other (Explain)

Who joined you: **Or Circle:** Ate Alone/Exercised Alone

Did you count calories eaten or expended? Yes No **Why?**

Meal/Snack location:

   Dining Table Restaurant In front of TV/Computer
   In bed Automobile Other (Explain)

Beverage Consumed:

   Soda Diet soda/seltzer water Tap/bottled water
   Milk/dairy alternative Other (Explain)

Reason for Eating:

   Nourishment Health Social Activity/Group Gathering
   Coping with feelings Controlling Emotions Other (Explain)

Reason for Exercise: (Check or circle the major reasons)

   Appearance/Weight Maintenance Fitness/Health Management
   Stress/Emotions/Mood or Feeling Management Socializing

At the beginning, during, or conclusion of the meal/snack/exercise, I felt: (Circle all that apply to any phase of this session)

Bad	Numb	Panic	Empowered	Distressed	Successful
Worried	Anxious	Sad	Depressed	Relief	Motivated
Fear	Lonely	Angry	Contempt	Calm	Self-Disciplined
Comfort	Misery	Control	Driven	Soothed	Traumatized
Shame	Guilt	Tired	Hungry	Other (List)	

Activity Reflection

Journal some thoughts about the meal or snack you selected or the exercise you undertook. Why did you select what you did? How did the choices relate to the rules, habits, and rituals your internal critic helped you set up?

Emotion Reflection

Journal about how the activity reflected the emotions you identified that went along with the activity. What brought the feelings/emotions on? Did they change during the session? What helped them change? Why did you select food/exercise as an outlet for those feelings?

When you complete your last session of Day 10, move on to the Phase One Reflection.

Phase One Session Log Sheet

Day 1 - Day 10

Complete the log for this food/exercise session. Place a checkmark next to or circle all that apply.

Date: **Day of Week:**   **Time:**   AM/PM

Reason for the session: Meal   Snack   Exercise   Other (Explain)

Who joined you: **Or Circle:**   Ate Alone/Exercised Alone

Did you count calories eaten or expended?   Yes   No   **Why?**

Meal/Snack location:

   Dining Table   Restaurant   In front of TV/Computer
   In bed   Automobile   Other (Explain)

Beverage Consumed:

   Soda   Diet soda/seltzer water   Tap/bottled water
   Milk/dairy alternative   Other (Explain)

Reason for Eating:

   Nourishment   Health   Social Activity/Group Gathering
   Coping with feelings   Controlling Emotions   Other (Explain)

Reason for Exercise: (Check or circle the major reasons)

   Appearance/Weight Maintenance   Fitness/Health Management
   Stress/Emotions/Mood or Feeling Management   Socializing

At the beginning, during, or conclusion of the meal/snack/exercise, I felt: (Circle all that apply to any phase of this session)

Bad	Numb	Panic	Empowered	Distressed	Successful
Worried	Anxious	Sad	Depressed	Relief	Motivated
Fear	Lonely	Angry	Contempt	Calm	Self-Disciplined
Comfort	Misery	Control	Driven	Soothed	Traumatized
Shame	Guilt	Tired	Hungry	Other (List)	

Activity Reflection

Journal some thoughts about the meal or snack you selected or the exercise you undertook. Why did you select what you did? How did the choices relate to the rules, habits, and rituals your internal critic helped you set up?

Emotion Reflection

Journal about how the activity reflected the emotions you identified that went along with the activity. What brought the feelings/emotions on? Did they change during the session? What helped them change? Why did you select food/exercise as an outlet for those feelings?

When you complete your last session of Day 10, move on to the Phase One Reflection.

Phase One Session Log Sheet

Day 1 - Day 10

Complete the log for this food/exercise session. Place a checkmark next to or circle all that apply.

Date: **Day of Week:** **Time:** AM/PM

Reason for the session: Meal Snack Exercise Other (Explain)

Who joined you: **Or Circle:** Ate Alone/Exercised Alone

Did you count calories eaten or expended? Yes No **Why?**

Meal/Snack location:

Dining Table	Restaurant	In front of TV/Computer
In bed	Automobile	Other (Explain)

Beverage Consumed:

Soda	Diet soda/seltzer water	Tap/bottled water
Milk/dairy alternative	Other (Explain)	

Reason for Eating:

Nourishment	Health	Social Activity/Group Gathering
Coping with feelings	Controlling Emotions	Other (Explain)

Reason for Exercise: (Check or circle the major reasons)

Appearance/Weight Maintenance	Fitness/Health Management
Stress/Emotions/Mood or Feeling Management	Socializing

At the beginning, during, or conclusion of the meal/snack/exercise, I felt: (Circle all that apply to any phase of this session)

Bad	Numb	Panic	Empowered	Distressed	Successful
Worried	Anxious	Sad	Depressed	Relief	Motivated
Fear	Lonely	Angry	Contempt	Calm	Self-Disciplined
Comfort	Misery	Control	Driven	Soothed	Traumatized
Shame	Guilt	Tired	Hungry	Other (List)	

ACTIVITY REFLECTION

Journal some thoughts about the meal or snack you selected or the exercise you undertook. Why did you select what you did? How did the choices relate to the rules, habits, and rituals your internal critic helped you set up?

EMOTION REFLECTION

Journal about how the activity reflected the emotions you identified that went along with the activity. What brought the feelings/emotions on? Did they change during the session? What helped them change? Why did you select food/exercise as an outlet for those feelings?

When you complete your last session of Day 10, move on to the Phase One Reflection.

Phase One Session Log Sheet

Day 1 - Day 10

Complete the log for this food/exercise session. Place a checkmark next to or circle all that apply.

Date:　　　　　　　　　**Day of Week:**　　　　　　　　　**Time:**　　　　AM/PM

Reason for the session:　　　Meal　　　　Snack　　　　Exercise　　　　Other (Explain)

Who joined you:　　　　　　　　**Or Circle:**　　　　　Ate Alone/Exercised Alone

Did you count calories eaten or expended?　　Yes　　　No　　**Why?**

Meal/Snack location:

Dining Table	Restaurant	In front of TV/Computer
In bed	Automobile	Other (Explain)

Beverage Consumed:

Soda	Diet soda/seltzer water	Tap/bottled water
Milk/dairy alternative	Other (Explain)	

Reason for Eating:

Nourishment	Health	Social Activity/Group Gathering
Coping with feelings	Controlling Emotions	Other (Explain)

Reason for Exercise: (Check or circle the major reasons)

Appearance/Weight Maintenance　　　　　　　　Fitness/Health Management
Stress/Emotions/Mood or Feeling Management　　Socializing

At the beginning, during, or conclusion of the meal/snack/exercise, I felt: (Circle all that apply to any phase of this session)

Bad	Numb	Panic	Empowered	Distressed	Successful
Worried	Anxious	Sad	Depressed	Relief	Motivated
Fear	Lonely	Angry	Contempt	Calm	Self-Disciplined
Comfort	Misery	Control	Driven	Soothed	Traumatized
Shame	Guilt	Tired	Hungry	Other (List)	

ACTIVITY REFLECTION

Journal some thoughts about the meal or snack you selected or the exercise you undertook. Why did you select what you did? How did the choices relate to the rules, habits, and rituals your internal critic helped you set up?

EMOTION REFLECTION

Journal about how the activity reflected the emotions you identified that went along with the activity. What brought the feelings/emotions on? Did they change during the session? What helped them change? Why did you select food/exercise as an outlet for those feelings?

When you complete your last session of Day 10, move on to the Phase One Reflection.

Phase One Session Log Sheet

Day 1 - Day 10

Complete the log for this food/exercise session. Place a checkmark next to or circle all that apply.

Date: **Day of Week:** **Time:** AM/PM

Reason for the session: Meal Snack Exercise Other (Explain)

Who joined you: **Or Circle:** Ate Alone/Exercised Alone

Did you count calories eaten or expended? Yes No **Why?**

Meal/Snack location:

Dining Table	Restaurant	In front of TV/Computer
In bed	Automobile	Other (Explain)

Beverage Consumed:

Soda	Diet soda/seltzer water	Tap/bottled water
Milk/dairy alternative	Other (Explain)	

Reason for Eating:

Nourishment	Health	Social Activity/Group Gathering
Coping with feelings	Controlling Emotions	Other (Explain)

Reason for Exercise: (Check or circle the major reasons)

Appearance/Weight Maintenance	Fitness/Health Management
Stress/Emotions/Mood or Feeling Management	Socializing

At the beginning, during, or conclusion of the meal/snack/exercise, I felt: (Circle all that apply to any phase of this session)

Bad	Numb	Panic	Empowered	Distressed	Successful
Worried	Anxious	Sad	Depressed	Relief	Motivated
Fear	Lonely	Angry	Contempt	Calm	Self-Disciplined
Comfort	Misery	Control	Driven	Soothed	Traumatized
Shame	Guilt	Tired	Hungry	Other (List)	

ACTIVITY REFLECTION

Journal some thoughts about the meal or snack you selected or the exercise you undertook. Why did you select what you did? How did the choices relate to the rules, habits, and rituals your internal critic helped you set up?

EMOTION REFLECTION

Journal about how the activity reflected the emotions you identified that went along with the activity. What brought the feelings/emotions on? Did they change during the session? What helped them change? Why did you select food/exercise as an outlet for those feelings?

When you complete your last session of Day 10, move on to the Phase One Reflection.

Phase One Session Log Sheet

Day 1 - Day 10

Complete the log for this food/exercise session. Place a checkmark next to or circle all that apply.

Date: **Day of Week:** **Time:** AM/PM

Reason for the session: Meal Snack Exercise Other (Explain)

Who joined you: **Or Circle:** Ate Alone/Exercised Alone

Did you count calories eaten or expended? Yes No **Why?**

Meal/Snack location:

Dining Table	Restaurant	In front of TV/Computer
In bed	Automobile	Other (Explain)

Beverage Consumed:

Soda	Diet soda/seltzer water	Tap/bottled water
Milk/dairy alternative	Other (Explain)	

Reason for Eating:

Nourishment	Health	Social Activity/Group Gathering
Coping with feelings	Controlling Emotions	Other (Explain)

Reason for Exercise: (Check or circle the major reasons)

Appearance/Weight Maintenance	Fitness/Health Management
Stress/Emotions/Mood or Feeling Management	Socializing

At the beginning, during, or conclusion of the meal/snack/exercise, I felt: (Circle all that apply to any phase of this session)

Bad	Numb	Panic	Empowered	Distressed	Successful
Worried	Anxious	Sad	Depressed	Relief	Motivated
Fear	Lonely	Angry	Contempt	Calm	Self-Disciplined
Comfort	Misery	Control	Driven	Soothed	Traumatized
Shame	Guilt	Tired	Hungry	Other (List)	

ACTIVITY REFLECTION

Journal some thoughts about the meal or snack you selected or the exercise you undertook. Why did you select what you did? How did the choices relate to the rules, habits, and rituals your internal critic helped you set up?

EMOTION REFLECTION

Journal about how the activity reflected the emotions you identified that went along with the activity. What brought the feelings/emotions on? Did they change during the session? What helped them change? Why did you select food/exercise as an outlet for those feelings?

When you complete your last session of Day 10, move on to the Phase One Reflection.

**If you need more pages for Phase One, you will find
an additional form to copy in the Appendix**

Phase One Reflection

Congratulations on completing the first phase of your mindfulness journey! Now it is time to look back at where you have been and take an honest look at the patterns that exist related to food and exercise. Find the patterns, tendencies, and emotional responses that tie together. You will need this awareness in order to begin making different cognitive choices moving forward.

Take a few moments to honestly answer the following questions:

On average, how many times did you eat a meal or snack each day? What was the average time interval between them? Did you skip meals? If so, why?

Did you notice any thoughts, emotions, feelings, or sensations between your meals and snacks? What were they? Describe them as completely as you can.

Did you ever go an entire day without eating? If so, why?

How many days did you exercise in the last ten days? If you didn't exercise at all, why?

What was the average duration of your exercise sessions? What were the primary reasons for exercise? How do those reasons relate to the emotions and feelings associated with them?

Did you have any days you exercised multiple times? If so, why?

Do you see any time patterns to your session timing? If so, what are they? If not, do you see any reason why the sessions may be so random?

Over the past ten days, what was the most common reason for your sessions? Nourishment, health, coping with feelings, controlling emotions, social gatherings, or other? Do you notice any patterns?

Who joined you most often or did you participate alone most often? Is there any relationship to feelings and emotions?

What were the top three to five most common feelings you experienced before, during, or after your sessions over the last ten days?

Reviewing the ACTIVITY REFLECTION journaling you completed after each session, what was the most common reason you selected the food or activities you did over the last ten days? What was the most observable relationship between the activities and the previously held rules, habits, and rituals you have?

Reviewing the EMOTION REFLECTION journaling you completed after each session, what brought the feelings/emotions on most frequently? Why did you select food/exercise as an outlet for those feelings most often?

In the last 10 days, have you engaged in any other emotional outlets besides food or exercise? (Examples might be shopping/money, sex/relationships, outbursts/emotions, alcohol/feelings etc.) If so, what are they and what were the emotions and situations that precipitated the response?

Food and exercise are two outlets used as coping tools instead of strictly for health or nourishment. You might have also identified some other emotional outlets that you practice as well. Take a few moments to brainstorm a long list of other, more life affirming, coping outlets that you could use instead. (Some ideas include but are not limited to: journaling, working a puzzle, spiritual practices like prayer/meditation, deep breathing, bathing/soaking, movie/favorite TV show, crafts, walking, music, dancing, etc.)

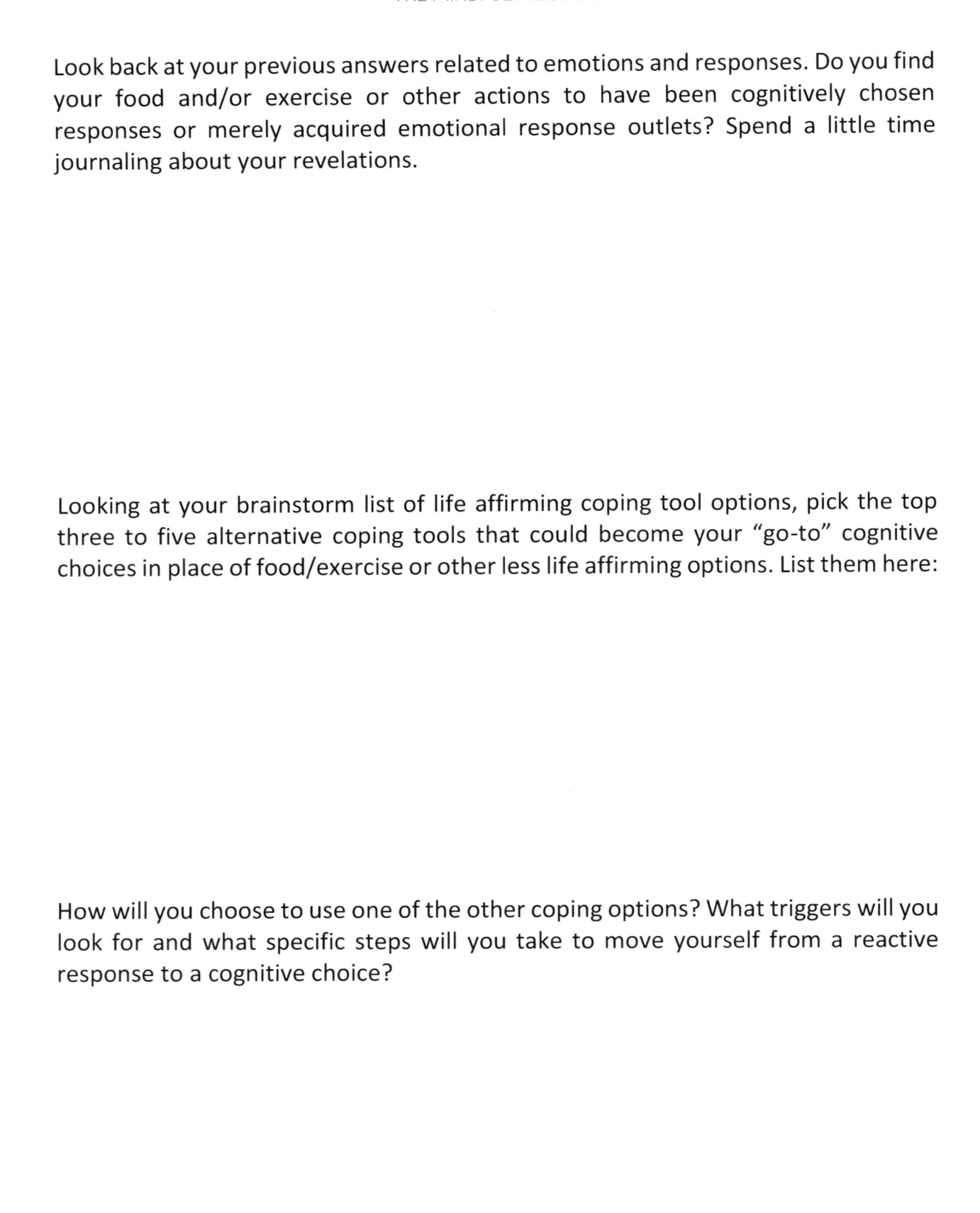

Look back at your previous answers related to emotions and responses. Do you find your food and/or exercise or other actions to have been cognitively chosen responses or merely acquired emotional response outlets? Spend a little time journaling about your revelations.

Looking at your brainstorm list of life affirming coping tool options, pick the top three to five alternative coping tools that could become your "go-to" cognitive choices in place of food/exercise or other less life affirming options. List them here:

How will you choose to use one of the other coping options? What triggers will you look for and what specific steps will you take to move yourself from a reactive response to a cognitive choice?

Phase Two

Out with the Old, In with the New

Hopefully over the last ten days you have increased your awareness of the "why" behind the "what" that surrounds your food and exercise choices. You have likely heard it said that we only have one body so we had better take care of it. However, many of the rules, habits, and rituals that have been created to manipulate and control food or exercise, do little to nourish and care for our bodies.

We each have an internal critic. However, how our internal critic came into being and how it became so loud and prominent is unique to each of us. How our internal critic began setting rules, placing compliance demands, and being overly critical of how we look and adhere to the rules and rituals is unique to us as well. When people battle other addictions and disorders like gambling, pornography, alcohol, or drugs, they are often advised to limit their environments to avoid temptations and triggers. This isn't the case with food and exercise. We need healthy foods to nourish our body and we need to exercise to maintain health and limit disease. When we begin to put self-control and positive self-talk into practice, the internal critic loses a foothold.

As you move into this next ten days, the focus will be on beginning to mindfully manage food and exercise choices. This mindful management allows you to begin noting the rules, habits, and rituals to allow you to consider other options. It also helps you begin to re-frame the way you cope with emotions and feelings. Taking the why's that you identify and find other ways to address them. This is an action oriented approach aimed at helping you find other self-controlled options and outlets. When you can successfully *pivot* and find other alternatives, food and exercise begin to come back in line with nourishment and health and move away from dieting and disorder.

There is a line between healthy exercise and nourishing food and abuse to our body. That line is individual for each one of us, but pretending that a line doesn't exist will prevent healing. You have to recognize and admit that you have an active role in placing and keeping food and exercise in their rightful place. Shifting your mindset from manipulating food or exercise to control weight or manage emotions and feelings toward maintaining or improving health is a big step forward. It is important to remember that learning new and different options and outlets doesn't mean the old rules, habits, and rituals go away. It will be a daily battle for you to consciously make self-controlled choices that move you in a new direction. Each small step you take moves you closer to new patterns that will become your new normal.

During the next ten days you will complete a session log for *each* food or exercise related activity you undertake just as you did over the last ten days. Ideally you will use a *new entry* for each session. However, if you do not have the time to commit to that level of discovery, doing one entry at the end of the day that captures the highlights is also an option. If you run out of session journal entry space before your last session on day 20, please go to the appendix section of the journal and make additional copies. If you get to your last session of day 20 and you aren't at the end of the provided Phase Two journaling pages, move on to the *Phase Two Reflection* activity. Once you have completed your last session on day 20, take some time to complete the Phase Two Reflection questions. Be sure to allow time to reflect and journal after *each* session as well as at the end of day 20.

Phase Two Session Log Sheet

Day 11 - Day 20

Complete the log for this food/exercise session. Place a checkmark next to or circle all that apply.

Date: **Day of Week:** **Time:** AM/PM

Reason for the session: Meal Snack Exercise Other (Explain)

Meal/Snack location:

Dining Table Restaurant In front of TV/Computer
In bed Automobile Other (Explain)

Beverage Consumed:

Soda Diet soda/seltzer water Tap/bottled water
Milk/dairy alternative Other (Explain)

Reason for Eating:

Nourishment Health Social Activity/Group Gathering
Coping with feelings Controlling Emotions Other (Explain)

Exercise Location and Activity:

Who joined you: **Or Circle:** Ate Alone/Exercised Alone

Reason for Exercise: (Check or circle the major reasons)

Appearance Fitness
Stress/Emotions/Mood Socializing

Did you count calories eaten or expended? Yes No **Why?**

List feelings experienced before/during/after:

How did you respond to those feelings?

Did you think about using an alternative coping tool?   Yes   No

Did you use an alternative coping tool? If so, what did you do and what happened?

What positive steps did you take to apply self-control to your food/exercise habits, rituals, routines at this session?

Activity Reflection

Journal some thoughts about the meal or snack you selected or the exercise you undertook. Why did you select what you did? Did you have control of your rules, habits, and rituals or did they have control of you?

Emotion Reflection

Journal about the feelings you experienced and how you responded to them. Could you have taken a breath and considered an alternative option? If you did consider and select an alternative, what led you to do that? What allowed you to be more aware of your feelings and responses? If you did not consider an alternative option, what got in the way?

When you complete your last session of Day 20, move on to the Phase Two Reflection.

Phase Two Session Log Sheet

Day 11 - Day 20

Complete the log for this food/exercise session. Place a checkmark next to or circle all that apply.

Date: **Day of Week:** **Time:** AM/PM

Reason for the session: Meal Snack Exercise Other (Explain)

Meal/Snack location:

    Dining Table Restaurant In front of TV/Computer
    In bed Automobile Other (Explain)

Beverage Consumed:

    Soda Diet soda/seltzer water Tap/bottled water
    Milk/dairy alternative Other (Explain)

Reason for Eating:

    Nourishment Health Social Activity/Group Gathering
    Coping with feelings Controlling Emotions Other (Explain)

Exercise Location and Activity:

Who joined you: **Or Circle:** Ate Alone/Exercised Alone

Reason for Exercise: (Check or circle the major reasons)

    Appearance Fitness
    Stress/Emotions/Mood Socializing

Did you count calories eaten or expended? Yes No **Why?**

List feelings experienced before/during/after:

How did you respond to those feelings?

Did you think about using an alternative coping tool?   Yes   No

Did you use an alternative coping tool? If so, what did you do and what happened?

What positive steps did you take to apply self-control to your food/exercise habits, rituals, routines at this session?

ACTIVITY REFLECTION

Journal some thoughts about the meal or snack you selected or the exercise you undertook. Why did you select what you did? Did you have control of your rules, habits, and rituals or did they have control of you?

EMOTION REFLECTION

Journal about the feelings you experienced and how you responded to them. Could you have taken a breath and considered an alternative option? If you did consider and select an alternative, what led you to do that? What allowed you to be more aware of your feelings and responses? If you did not consider an alternative option, what got in the way?

When you complete your last session of Day 20, move on to the Phase Two Reflection.

Phase Two Session Log Sheet

Day 11 - Day 20

Complete the log for this food/exercise session. Place a checkmark next to or circle all that apply.

Date: **Day of Week**:   **Time**:   AM/PM

Reason for the session: Meal   Snack   Exercise   Other (Explain)

Meal/Snack location:

    Dining Table   Restaurant   In front of TV/Computer
    In bed   Automobile   Other (Explain)

Beverage Consumed:

    Soda   Diet soda/seltzer water   Tap/bottled water
    Milk/dairy alternative   Other (Explain)

Reason for Eating:

    Nourishment   Health   Social Activity/Group Gathering
    Coping with feelings   Controlling Emotions   Other (Explain)

Exercise Location and Activity:

Who joined you: **Or Circle**:   Ate Alone/Exercised Alone

Reason for Exercise: (Check or circle the major reasons)

    Appearance   Fitness
    Stress/Emotions/Mood   Socializing

Did you count calories eaten or expended?   Yes   No   **Why?**

List feelings experienced before/during/after:

How did you respond to those feelings?

Did you think about using an alternative coping tool?   Yes   No

Did you use an alternative coping tool? If so, what did you do and what happened?

What positive steps did you take to apply self-control to your food/exercise habits, rituals, routines at this session?

Activity Reflection

Journal some thoughts about the meal or snack you selected or the exercise you undertook. Why did you select what you did? Did you have control of your rules, habits, and rituals or did they have control of you?

Emotion Reflection

Journal about the feelings you experienced and how you responded to them. Could you have taken a breath and considered an alternative option? If you did consider and select an alternative, what led you to do that? What allowed you to be more aware of your feelings and responses? If you did not consider an alternative option, what got in the way?

When you complete your last session of Day 20, move on to the Phase Two Reflection.

Phase Two Session Log Sheet

Day 11 - Day 20

Complete the log for this food/exercise session. Place a checkmark next to or circle all that apply.

Date: **Day of Week:** **Time:** AM/PM

Reason for the session: Meal Snack Exercise Other (Explain)

Meal/Snack location:

    Dining Table Restaurant In front of TV/Computer
    In bed Automobile Other (Explain)

Beverage Consumed:

    Soda Diet soda/seltzer water Tap/bottled water
    Milk/dairy alternative Other (Explain)

Reason for Eating:

    Nourishment Health Social Activity/Group Gathering
    Coping with feelings Controlling Emotions Other (Explain)

Exercise Location and Activity:

Who joined you: **Or Circle:** Ate Alone/Exercised Alone

Reason for Exercise: (Check or circle the major reasons)

    Appearance Fitness
    Stress/Emotions/Mood Socializing

Did you count calories eaten or expended? Yes No **Why?**

List feelings experienced before/during/after:

How did you respond to those feelings?

Did you think about using an alternative coping tool?   Yes   No

Did you use an alternative coping tool? If so, what did you do and what happened?

What positive steps did you take to apply self-control to your food/exercise habits, rituals, routines at this session?

Activity Reflection

Journal some thoughts about the meal or snack you selected or the exercise you undertook. Why did you select what you did? Did you have control of your rules, habits, and rituals or did they have control of you?

Emotion Reflection

Journal about the feelings you experienced and how you responded to them. Could you have taken a breath and considered an alternative option? If you did consider and select an alternative, what led you to do that? What allowed you to be more aware of your feelings and responses? If you did not consider an alternative option, what got in the way?

When you complete your last session of Day 20, move on to the Phase Two Reflection.

Phase Two Session Log Sheet

Day 11 - Day 20

Complete the log for this food/exercise session. Place a checkmark next to or circle all that apply.

Date: **Day of Week:** **Time:** AM/PM

Reason for the session: Meal Snack Exercise Other (Explain)

Meal/Snack location:

Dining Table Restaurant In front of TV/Computer
In bed Automobile Other (Explain)

Beverage Consumed:

Soda Diet soda/seltzer water Tap/bottled water
Milk/dairy alternative Other (Explain)

Reason for Eating:

Nourishment Health Social Activity/Group Gathering
Coping with feelings Controlling Emotions Other (Explain)

Exercise Location and Activity:

Who joined you: **Or Circle:** Ate Alone/Exercised Alone

Reason for Exercise: (Check or circle the major reasons)

Appearance Fitness
Stress/Emotions/Mood Socializing

Did you count calories eaten or expended? Yes No **Why?**

List feelings experienced before/during/after:

How did you respond to those feelings?

Did you think about using an alternative coping tool? Yes No

Did you use an alternative coping tool? If so, what did you do and what happened?

What positive steps did you take to apply self-control to your food/exercise habits, rituals, routines at this session?

Activity Reflection

Journal some thoughts about the meal or snack you selected or the exercise you undertook. Why did you select what you did? Did you have control of your rules, habits, and rituals or did they have control of you?

Emotion Reflection

Journal about the feelings you experienced and how you responded to them. Could you have taken a breath and considered an alternative option? If you did consider and select an alternative, what led you to do that? What allowed you to be more aware of your feelings and responses? If you did not consider an alternative option, what got in the way?

When you complete your last session of Day 20, move on to the Phase Two Reflection.

Phase Two Session Log Sheet

Day 11 - Day 20

Complete the log for this food/exercise session. Place a checkmark next to or circle all that apply.

Date:　　　　　　　　**Day of Week:**　　　　　　　　**Time:**　　　　AM/PM

Reason for the session:　　Meal　　　　Snack　　　　Exercise　　　　Other (Explain)

Meal/Snack location:

　　Dining Table　　　　Restaurant　　　　　　　　In front of TV/Computer
　　In bed　　　　　　　Automobile　　　　　　　　Other (Explain)

Beverage Consumed:

　　Soda　　　　　　　　　　Diet soda/seltzer water　　　　Tap/bottled water
　　Milk/dairy alternative　　Other (Explain)

Reason for Eating:

　　Nourishment　　　　　Health　　　　　　　　　Social Activity/Group Gathering
　　Coping with feelings　Controlling Emotions　　Other (Explain)

Exercise Location and Activity:

Who joined you:　　　　　　　　　**Or Circle:**　　　　Ate Alone/Exercised Alone

Reason for Exercise: (Check or circle the major reasons)

　　Appearance　　　　　　　　　　Fitness
　　Stress/Emotions/Mood　　　　　Socializing

Did you count calories eaten or expended?　　Yes　　No　　**Why?**

List feelings experienced before/during/after:

How did you respond to those feelings?

Did you think about using an alternative coping tool?   Yes   No

Did you use an alternative coping tool? If so, what did you do and what happened?

What positive steps did you take to apply self-control to your food/exercise habits, rituals, routines at this session?

Activity Reflection

Journal some thoughts about the meal or snack you selected or the exercise you undertook. Why did you select what you did? Did you have control of your rules, habits, and rituals or did they have control of you?

Emotion Reflection

Journal about the feelings you experienced and how you responded to them. Could you have taken a breath and considered an alternative option? If you did consider and select an alternative, what led you to do that? What allowed you to be more aware of your feelings and responses? If you did not consider an alternative option, what got in the way?

When you complete your last session of Day 20, move on to the Phase Two Reflection.

Phase Two Session Log Sheet

Day 11 - Day 20

Complete the log for this food/exercise session. Place a checkmark next to or circle all that apply.

Date: **Day of Week:** **Time:** AM/PM

Reason for the session: Meal Snack Exercise Other (Explain)

Meal/Snack location:

    Dining Table Restaurant In front of TV/Computer
    In bed Automobile Other (Explain)

Beverage Consumed:

    Soda Diet soda/seltzer water Tap/bottled water
    Milk/dairy alternative Other (Explain)

Reason for Eating:

    Nourishment Health Social Activity/Group Gathering
    Coping with feelings Controlling Emotions Other (Explain)

Exercise Location and Activity:

Who joined you: **Or Circle:** Ate Alone/Exercised Alone

Reason for Exercise: (Check or circle the major reasons)

    Appearance Fitness
    Stress/Emotions/Mood Socializing

Did you count calories eaten or expended? Yes No **Why?**

List feelings experienced before/during/after:

How did you respond to those feelings?

Did you think about using an alternative coping tool?   Yes   No

Did you use an alternative coping tool? If so, what did you do and what happened?

What positive steps did you take to apply self-control to your food/exercise habits, rituals, routines at this session?

Activity Reflection

Journal some thoughts about the meal or snack you selected or the exercise you undertook. Why did you select what you did? Did you have control of your rules, habits, and rituals or did they have control of you?

Emotion Reflection

Journal about the feelings you experienced and how you responded to them. Could you have taken a breath and considered an alternative option? If you did consider and select an alternative, what led you to do that? What allowed you to be more aware of your feelings and responses? If you did not consider an alternative option, what got in the way?

When you complete your last session of Day 20, move on to the Phase Two Reflection.

Phase Two Session Log Sheet

Day 11 - Day 20

Complete the log for this food/exercise session. Place a checkmark next to or circle all that apply.

Date: **Day of Week:**   **Time:**   AM/PM

Reason for the session: Meal   Snack   Exercise   Other (Explain)

Meal/Snack location:

    Dining Table   Restaurant   In front of TV/Computer
    In bed   Automobile   Other (Explain)

Beverage Consumed:

    Soda   Diet soda/seltzer water   Tap/bottled water
    Milk/dairy alternative   Other (Explain)

Reason for Eating:

    Nourishment   Health   Social Activity/Group Gathering
    Coping with feelings   Controlling Emotions   Other (Explain)

Exercise Location and Activity:

Who joined you: **Or Circle:**   Ate Alone/Exercised Alone

Reason for Exercise: (Check or circle the major reasons)

    Appearance   Fitness
    Stress/Emotions/Mood   Socializing

Did you count calories eaten or expended?   Yes   No   **Why?**

List feelings experienced before/during/after:

How did you respond to those feelings?

Did you think about using an alternative coping tool?   Yes   No

Did you use an alternative coping tool? If so, what did you do and what happened?

What positive steps did you take to apply self-control to your food/exercise habits, rituals, routines at this session?

ACTIVITY REFLECTION

Journal some thoughts about the meal or snack you selected or the exercise you undertook. Why did you select what you did? Did you have control of your rules, habits, and rituals or did they have control of you?

EMOTION REFLECTION

Journal about the feelings you experienced and how you responded to them. Could you have taken a breath and considered an alternative option? If you did consider and select an alternative, what led you to do that? What allowed you to be more aware of your feelings and responses? If you did not consider an alternative option, what got in the way?

When you complete your last session of Day 20, move on to the Phase Two Reflection.

Phase Two Session Log Sheet

Day 11 - Day 20

Complete the log for this food/exercise session. Place a checkmark next to or circle all that apply.

Date: **Day of Week:**   **Time:**   AM/PM

Reason for the session: Meal   Snack   Exercise   Other (Explain)

Meal/Snack location:

     Dining Table   Restaurant   In front of TV/Computer
     In bed   Automobile   Other (Explain)

Beverage Consumed:

     Soda   Diet soda/seltzer water   Tap/bottled water
     Milk/dairy alternative   Other (Explain)

Reason for Eating:

     Nourishment   Health   Social Activity/Group Gathering
     Coping with feelings   Controlling Emotions   Other (Explain)

Exercise Location and Activity:

Who joined you: **Or Circle:**   Ate Alone/Exercised Alone

Reason for Exercise: (Check or circle the major reasons)

     Appearance   Fitness
     Stress/Emotions/Mood   Socializing

Did you count calories eaten or expended?   Yes   No   **Why?**

List feelings experienced before/during/after:

How did you respond to those feelings?

Did you think about using an alternative coping tool?   Yes   No

Did you use an alternative coping tool? If so, what did you do and what happened?

What positive steps did you take to apply self-control to your food/exercise habits, rituals, routines at this session?

Activity Reflection

Journal some thoughts about the meal or snack you selected or the exercise you undertook. Why did you select what you did? Did you have control of your rules, habits, and rituals or did they have control of you?

Emotion Reflection

Journal about the feelings you experienced and how you responded to them. Could you have taken a breath and considered an alternative option? If you did consider and select an alternative, what led you to do that? What allowed you to be more aware of your feelings and responses? If you did not consider an alternative option, what got in the way?

When you complete your last session of Day 20, move on to the Phase Two Reflection.

Phase Two Session Log Sheet

Day 11 - Day 20

Complete the log for this food/exercise session. Place a checkmark next to or circle all that apply.

Date: **Day of Week:**   **Time:**   AM/PM

Reason for the session: Meal   Snack   Exercise   Other (Explain)

Meal/Snack location:

    Dining Table   Restaurant   In front of TV/Computer
    In bed   Automobile   Other (Explain)

Beverage Consumed:

    Soda   Diet soda/seltzer water   Tap/bottled water
    Milk/dairy alternative   Other (Explain)

Reason for Eating:

    Nourishment   Health   Social Activity/Group Gathering
    Coping with feelings   Controlling Emotions   Other (Explain)

Exercise Location and Activity:

Who joined you: **Or Circle:**   Ate Alone/Exercised Alone

Reason for Exercise: (Check or circle the major reasons)

    Appearance   Fitness
    Stress/Emotions/Mood   Socializing

Did you count calories eaten or expended?   Yes   No   **Why?**

List feelings experienced before/during/after:

How did you respond to those feelings?

Did you think about using an alternative coping tool?   Yes   No

Did you use an alternative coping tool? If so, what did you do and what happened?

What positive steps did you take to apply self-control to your food/exercise habits, rituals, routines at this session?

ACTIVITY REFLECTION

Journal some thoughts about the meal or snack you selected or the exercise you undertook. Why did you select what you did? Did you have control of your rules, habits, and rituals or did they have control of you?

EMOTION REFLECTION

Journal about the feelings you experienced and how you responded to them. Could you have taken a breath and considered an alternative option? If you did consider and select an alternative, what led you to do that? What allowed you to be more aware of your feelings and responses? If you did not consider an alternative option, what got in the way?

When you complete your last session of Day 20, move on to the Phase Two Reflection.

Phase Two Session Log Sheet

Day 11 - Day 20

Complete the log for this food/exercise session. Place a checkmark next to or circle all that apply.

Date: **Day of Week:** **Time:** AM/PM

Reason for the session: Meal Snack Exercise Other (Explain)

Meal/Snack location:

Dining Table Restaurant In front of TV/Computer
In bed Automobile Other (Explain)

Beverage Consumed:

Soda Diet soda/seltzer water Tap/bottled water
Milk/dairy alternative Other (Explain)

Reason for Eating:

Nourishment Health Social Activity/Group Gathering
Coping with feelings Controlling Emotions Other (Explain)

Exercise Location and Activity:

Who joined you: **Or Circle:** Ate Alone/Exercised Alone

Reason for Exercise: (Check or circle the major reasons)

Appearance Fitness
Stress/Emotions/Mood Socializing

Did you count calories eaten or expended? Yes No **Why?**

List feelings experienced before/during/after:

How did you respond to those feelings?

Did you think about using an alternative coping tool?   Yes   No

Did you use an alternative coping tool? If so, what did you do and what happened?

What positive steps did you take to apply self-control to your food/exercise habits, rituals, routines at this session?

Activity Reflection

Journal some thoughts about the meal or snack you selected or the exercise you undertook. Why did you select what you did? Did you have control of your rules, habits, and rituals or did they have control of you?

Emotion Reflection

Journal about the feelings you experienced and how you responded to them. Could you have taken a breath and considered an alternative option? If you did consider and select an alternative, what led you to do that? What allowed you to be more aware of your feelings and responses? If you did not consider an alternative option, what got in the way?

When you complete your last session of Day 20, move on to the Phase Two Reflection.

Phase Two Session Log Sheet

Day 11 - Day 20

Complete the log for this food/exercise session. Place a checkmark next to or circle all that apply.

Date: **Day of Week:**   **Time:**   AM/PM

Reason for the session: Meal   Snack   Exercise   Other (Explain)

Meal/Snack location:

   Dining Table   Restaurant   In front of TV/Computer
   In bed   Automobile   Other (Explain)

Beverage Consumed:

   Soda   Diet soda/seltzer water   Tap/bottled water
   Milk/dairy alternative   Other (Explain)

Reason for Eating:

   Nourishment   Health   Social Activity/Group Gathering
   Coping with feelings   Controlling Emotions   Other (Explain)

Exercise Location and Activity:

Who joined you: **Or Circle:**   Ate Alone/Exercised Alone

Reason for Exercise: (Check or circle the major reasons)

   Appearance   Fitness
   Stress/Emotions/Mood   Socializing

Did you count calories eaten or expended?   Yes   No   **Why?**

List feelings experienced before/during/after:

How did you respond to those feelings?

Did you think about using an alternative coping tool?   Yes   No

Did you use an alternative coping tool? If so, what did you do and what happened?

What positive steps did you take to apply self-control to your food/exercise habits, rituals, routines at this session?

Activity Reflection

Journal some thoughts about the meal or snack you selected or the exercise you undertook. Why did you select what you did? Did you have control of your rules, habits, and rituals or did they have control of you?

Emotion Reflection

Journal about the feelings you experienced and how you responded to them. Could you have taken a breath and considered an alternative option? If you did consider and select an alternative, what led you to do that? What allowed you to be more aware of your feelings and responses? If you did not consider an alternative option, what got in the way?

When you complete your last session of Day 20, move on to the Phase Two Reflection.

Phase Two Session Log Sheet

Day 11 - Day 20

Complete the log for this food/exercise session. Place a checkmark next to or circle all that apply.

Date: **Day of Week:**   **Time:**   AM/PM

Reason for the session: Meal   Snack   Exercise   Other (Explain)

Meal/Snack location:

   Dining Table   Restaurant   In front of TV/Computer
   In bed   Automobile   Other (Explain)

Beverage Consumed:

   Soda   Diet soda/seltzer water   Tap/bottled water
   Milk/dairy alternative   Other (Explain)

Reason for Eating:

   Nourishment   Health   Social Activity/Group Gathering
   Coping with feelings   Controlling Emotions   Other (Explain)

Exercise Location and Activity:

Who joined you: **Or Circle:**   Ate Alone/Exercised Alone

Reason for Exercise: (Check or circle the major reasons)

   Appearance   Fitness
   Stress/Emotions/Mood   Socializing

Did you count calories eaten or expended?   Yes   No   **Why?**

List feelings experienced before/during/after:

How did you respond to those feelings?

Did you think about using an alternative coping tool?   Yes   No

Did you use an alternative coping tool? If so, what did you do and what happened?

What positive steps did you take to apply self-control to your food/exercise habits, rituals, routines at this session?

ACTIVITY REFLECTION

Journal some thoughts about the meal or snack you selected or the exercise you undertook. Why did you select what you did? Did you have control of your rules, habits, and rituals or did they have control of you?

EMOTION REFLECTION

Journal about the feelings you experienced and how you responded to them. Could you have taken a breath and considered an alternative option? If you did consider and select an alternative, what led you to do that? What allowed you to be more aware of your feelings and responses? If you did not consider an alternative option, what got in the way?

When you complete your last session of Day 20, move on to the Phase Two Reflection.

Phase Two Session Log Sheet

Day 11 - Day 20

Complete the log for this food/exercise session. Place a checkmark next to or circle all that apply.

Date:　　　　　　　　**Day of Week:**　　　　　　　**Time:**　　　　AM/PM

Reason for the session:　　Meal　　　　Snack　　　　Exercise　　　　Other (Explain)

Meal/Snack location:

　　Dining Table　　　　　Restaurant　　　　　　　　In front of TV/Computer
　　In bed　　　　　　　　Automobile　　　　　　　　Other (Explain)

Beverage Consumed:

　　Soda　　　　　　　　　Diet soda/seltzer water　　Tap/bottled water
　　Milk/dairy alternative　Other (Explain)

Reason for Eating:

　　Nourishment　　　　　Health　　　　　　　　　　Social Activity/Group Gathering
　　Coping with feelings　Controlling Emotions　　　Other (Explain)

Exercise Location and Activity:

Who joined you:　　　　　　　　　　**Or Circle:**　　　Ate Alone/Exercised Alone

Reason for Exercise: (Check or circle the major reasons)

　　Appearance　　　　　　　　　　Fitness
　　Stress/Emotions/Mood　　　　　Socializing

Did you count calories eaten or expended?　　Yes　　　No　　　**Why?**

List feelings experienced before/during/after:

How did you respond to those feelings?

Did you think about using an alternative coping tool?   Yes   No

Did you use an alternative coping tool? If so, what did you do and what happened?

What positive steps did you take to apply self-control to your food/exercise habits, rituals, routines at this session?

Activity Reflection

Journal some thoughts about the meal or snack you selected or the exercise you undertook. Why did you select what you did? Did you have control of your rules, habits, and rituals or did they have control of you?

Emotion Reflection

Journal about the feelings you experienced and how you responded to them. Could you have taken a breath and considered an alternative option? If you did consider and select an alternative, what led you to do that? What allowed you to be more aware of your feelings and responses? If you did not consider an alternative option, what got in the way?

When you complete your last session of Day 20, move on to the Phase Two Reflection.

Phase Two Session Log Sheet

Day 11 - Day 20

Complete the log for this food/exercise session. Place a checkmark next to or circle all that apply.

Date: **Day of Week:**   **Time:**   AM/PM

Reason for the session: Meal   Snack   Exercise   Other (Explain)

Meal/Snack location:

    Dining Table   Restaurant   In front of TV/Computer
    In bed   Automobile   Other (Explain)

Beverage Consumed:

    Soda   Diet soda/seltzer water   Tap/bottled water
    Milk/dairy alternative   Other (Explain)

Reason for Eating:

    Nourishment   Health   Social Activity/Group Gathering
    Coping with feelings   Controlling Emotions   Other (Explain)

Exercise Location and Activity:

Who joined you: **Or Circle:**   Ate Alone/Exercised Alone

Reason for Exercise: (Check or circle the major reasons)

    Appearance   Fitness
    Stress/Emotions/Mood   Socializing

Did you count calories eaten or expended?   Yes   No   **Why?**

List feelings experienced before/during/after:

How did you respond to those feelings?

Did you think about using an alternative coping tool?   Yes   No

Did you use an alternative coping tool? If so, what did you do and what happened?

What positive steps did you take to apply self-control to your food/exercise habits, rituals, routines at this session?

Activity Reflection

Journal some thoughts about the meal or snack you selected or the exercise you undertook. Why did you select what you did? Did you have control of your rules, habits, and rituals or did they have control of you?

Emotion Reflection

Journal about the feelings you experienced and how you responded to them. Could you have taken a breath and considered an alternative option? If you did consider and select an alternative, what led you to do that? What allowed you to be more aware of your feelings and responses? If you did not consider an alternative option, what got in the way?

When you complete your last session of Day 20, move on to the Phase Two Reflection.

Phase Two Session Log Sheet

Day 11 - Day 20

Complete the log for this food/exercise session. Place a checkmark next to or circle all that apply.

Date: **Day of Week:** **Time:** AM/PM

Reason for the session: Meal Snack Exercise Other (Explain)

Meal/Snack location:

Dining Table	Restaurant	In front of TV/Computer
In bed	Automobile	Other (Explain)

Beverage Consumed:

Soda	Diet soda/seltzer water	Tap/bottled water
Milk/dairy alternative	Other (Explain)	

Reason for Eating:

Nourishment	Health	Social Activity/Group Gathering
Coping with feelings	Controlling Emotions	Other (Explain)

Exercise Location and Activity:

Who joined you: **Or Circle:** Ate Alone/Exercised Alone

Reason for Exercise: (Check or circle the major reasons)

Appearance	Fitness
Stress/Emotions/Mood	Socializing

Did you count calories eaten or expended? Yes No **Why?**

List feelings experienced before/during/after:

How did you respond to those feelings?

Did you think about using an alternative coping tool?   Yes   No

Did you use an alternative coping tool? If so, what did you do and what happened?

What positive steps did you take to apply self-control to your food/exercise habits, rituals, routines at this session?

Activity Reflection

Journal some thoughts about the meal or snack you selected or the exercise you undertook. Why did you select what you did? Did you have control of your rules, habits, and rituals or did they have control of you?

Emotion Reflection

Journal about the feelings you experienced and how you responded to them. Could you have taken a breath and considered an alternative option? If you did consider and select an alternative, what led you to do that? What allowed you to be more aware of your feelings and responses? If you did not consider an alternative option, what got in the way?

When you complete your last session of Day 20, move on to the Phase Two Reflection.

Phase Two Session Log Sheet

Day 11 - Day 20

Complete the log for this food/exercise session. Place a checkmark next to or circle all that apply.

Date: **Day of Week:**   **Time:**   AM/PM

Reason for the session: Meal   Snack   Exercise   Other (Explain)

Meal/Snack location:

   Dining Table   Restaurant   In front of TV/Computer
   In bed   Automobile   Other (Explain)

Beverage Consumed:

   Soda   Diet soda/seltzer water   Tap/bottled water
   Milk/dairy alternative Other (Explain)

Reason for Eating:

   Nourishment   Health   Social Activity/Group Gathering
   Coping with feelings   Controlling Emotions   Other (Explain)

Exercise Location and Activity:

Who joined you: **Or Circle:**   Ate Alone/Exercised Alone

Reason for Exercise: (Check or circle the major reasons)

   Appearance   Fitness
   Stress/Emotions/Mood   Socializing

Did you count calories eaten or expended?   Yes   No   **Why?**

List feelings experienced before/during/after:

How did you respond to those feelings?

Did you think about using an alternative coping tool? Yes No

Did you use an alternative coping tool? If so, what did you do and what happened?

What positive steps did you take to apply self-control to your food/exercise habits, rituals, routines at this session?

ACTIVITY REFLECTION

Journal some thoughts about the meal or snack you selected or the exercise you undertook. Why did you select what you did? Did you have control of your rules, habits, and rituals or did they have control of you?

EMOTION REFLECTION

Journal about the feelings you experienced and how you responded to them. Could you have taken a breath and considered an alternative option? If you did consider and select an alternative, what led you to do that? What allowed you to be more aware of your feelings and responses? If you did not consider an alternative option, what got in the way?

When you complete your last session of Day 20, move on to the Phase Two Reflection.

Phase Two Session Log Sheet

Day 11 - Day 20

Complete the log for this food/exercise session. Place a checkmark next to or circle all that apply.

Date: **Day of Week:** **Time:** AM/PM

Reason for the session: Meal Snack Exercise Other (Explain)

Meal/Snack location:

Dining Table	Restaurant	In front of TV/Computer
In bed	Automobile	Other (Explain)

Beverage Consumed:

Soda	Diet soda/seltzer water	Tap/bottled water
Milk/dairy alternative	Other (Explain)	

Reason for Eating:

Nourishment	Health	Social Activity/Group Gathering
Coping with feelings	Controlling Emotions	Other (Explain)

Exercise Location and Activity:

Who joined you: **Or Circle:** Ate Alone/Exercised Alone

Reason for Exercise: (Check or circle the major reasons)

Appearance	Fitness
Stress/Emotions/Mood	Socializing

Did you count calories eaten or expended? Yes No **Why?**

List feelings experienced before/during/after:

How did you respond to those feelings?

Did you think about using an alternative coping tool?   Yes   No

Did you use an alternative coping tool? If so, what did you do and what happened?

What positive steps did you take to apply self-control to your food/exercise habits, rituals, routines at this session?

Activity Reflection

Journal some thoughts about the meal or snack you selected or the exercise you undertook. Why did you select what you did? Did you have control of your rules, habits, and rituals or did they have control of you?

Emotion Reflection

Journal about the feelings you experienced and how you responded to them. Could you have taken a breath and considered an alternative option? If you did consider and select an alternative, what led you to do that? What allowed you to be more aware of your feelings and responses? If you did not consider an alternative option, what got in the way?

When you complete your last session of Day 20, move on to the Phase Two Reflection.

Phase Two Session Log Sheet

Day 11 - Day 20

Complete the log for this food/exercise session. Place a checkmark next to or circle all that apply.

Date: **Day of Week:** **Time:** AM/PM

Reason for the session: Meal Snack Exercise Other (Explain)

Meal/Snack location:

    Dining Table Restaurant In front of TV/Computer
    In bed Automobile Other (Explain)

Beverage Consumed:

    Soda Diet soda/seltzer water Tap/bottled water
    Milk/dairy alternative Other (Explain)

Reason for Eating:

    Nourishment Health Social Activity/Group Gathering
    Coping with feelings Controlling Emotions Other (Explain)

Exercise Location and Activity:

Who joined you: **Or Circle:** Ate Alone/Exercised Alone

Reason for Exercise: (Check or circle the major reasons)

    Appearance Fitness
    Stress/Emotions/Mood Socializing

Did you count calories eaten or expended? Yes No **Why?**

List feelings experienced before/during/after:

How did you respond to those feelings?

Did you think about using an alternative coping tool?   Yes   No

Did you use an alternative coping tool? If so, what did you do and what happened?

What positive steps did you take to apply self-control to your food/exercise habits, rituals, routines at this session?

Activity Reflection

Journal some thoughts about the meal or snack you selected or the exercise you undertook. Why did you select what you did? Did you have control of your rules, habits, and rituals or did they have control of you?

Emotion Reflection

Journal about the feelings you experienced and how you responded to them. Could you have taken a breath and considered an alternative option? If you did consider and select an alternative, what led you to do that? What allowed you to be more aware of your feelings and responses? If you did not consider an alternative option, what got in the way?

When you complete your last session of Day 20, move on to the Phase Two Reflection.

Phase Two Session Log Sheet

Day 11 - Day 20

Complete the log for this food/exercise session. Place a checkmark next to or circle all that apply.

Date: **Day of Week:**   **Time:**   AM/PM

Reason for the session: Meal   Snack   Exercise   Other (Explain)

Meal/Snack location:

    Dining Table   Restaurant   In front of TV/Computer
    In bed   Automobile   Other (Explain)

Beverage Consumed:

    Soda   Diet soda/seltzer water   Tap/bottled water
    Milk/dairy alternative   Other (Explain)

Reason for Eating:

    Nourishment   Health   Social Activity/Group Gathering
    Coping with feelings   Controlling Emotions   Other (Explain)

Exercise Location and Activity:

Who joined you: **Or Circle:**   Ate Alone/Exercised Alone

Reason for Exercise: (Check or circle the major reasons)

    Appearance   Fitness
    Stress/Emotions/Mood   Socializing

Did you count calories eaten or expended?   Yes   No   **Why?**

List feelings experienced before/during/after:

How did you respond to those feelings?

Did you think about using an alternative coping tool?   Yes   No

Did you use an alternative coping tool? If so, what did you do and what happened?

What positive steps did you take to apply self-control to your food/exercise habits, rituals, routines at this session?

Activity Reflection

Journal some thoughts about the meal or snack you selected or the exercise you undertook. Why did you select what you did? Did you have control of your rules, habits, and rituals or did they have control of you?

Emotion Reflection

Journal about the feelings you experienced and how you responded to them. Could you have taken a breath and considered an alternative option? If you did consider and select an alternative, what led you to do that? What allowed you to be more aware of your feelings and responses? If you did not consider an alternative option, what got in the way?

When you complete your last session of Day 20, move on to the Phase Two Reflection.

Phase Two Session Log Sheet

Day 11 - Day 20

Complete the log for this food/exercise session. Place a checkmark next to or circle all that apply.

Date: **Day of Week:** **Time:** AM/PM

Reason for the session: Meal Snack Exercise Other (Explain)

Meal/Snack location:

> Dining Table Restaurant In front of TV/Computer
> In bed Automobile Other (Explain)

Beverage Consumed:

> Soda Diet soda/seltzer water Tap/bottled water
> Milk/dairy alternative Other (Explain)

Reason for Eating:

> Nourishment Health Social Activity/Group Gathering
> Coping with feelings Controlling Emotions Other (Explain)

Exercise Location and Activity:

Who joined you: **Or Circle:** Ate Alone/Exercised Alone

Reason for Exercise: (Check or circle the major reasons)

> Appearance Fitness
> Stress/Emotions/Mood Socializing

Did you count calories eaten or expended? Yes No **Why?**

List feelings experienced before/during/after:

How did you respond to those feelings?

Did you think about using an alternative coping tool?   Yes   No

Did you use an alternative coping tool? If so, what did you do and what happened?

What positive steps did you take to apply self-control to your food/exercise habits, rituals, routines at this session?

Activity Reflection

Journal some thoughts about the meal or snack you selected or the exercise you undertook. Why did you select what you did? Did you have control of your rules, habits, and rituals or did they have control of you?

Emotion Reflection

Journal about the feelings you experienced and how you responded to them. Could you have taken a breath and considered an alternative option? If you did consider and select an alternative, what led you to do that? What allowed you to be more aware of your feelings and responses? If you did not consider an alternative option, what got in the way?

When you complete your last session of Day 20, move on to the Phase Two Reflection.

Phase Two Session Log Sheet

Day 11 - Day 20

Complete the log for this food/exercise session. Place a checkmark next to or circle all that apply.

Date: **Day of Week:**   **Time:**   AM/PM

Reason for the session: Meal   Snack   Exercise   Other (Explain)

Meal/Snack location:

Dining Table	Restaurant	In front of TV/Computer
In bed	Automobile	Other (Explain)

Beverage Consumed:

Soda	Diet soda/seltzer water	Tap/bottled water
Milk/dairy alternative	Other (Explain)	

Reason for Eating:

Nourishment	Health	Social Activity/Group Gathering
Coping with feelings	Controlling Emotions	Other (Explain)

Exercise Location and Activity:

Who joined you: **Or Circle:**   Ate Alone/Exercised Alone

Reason for Exercise: (Check or circle the major reasons)

Appearance	Fitness
Stress/Emotions/Mood	Socializing

Did you count calories eaten or expended?   Yes   No   **Why?**

List feelings experienced before/during/after:

How did you respond to those feelings?

Did you think about using an alternative coping tool?   Yes   No

Did you use an alternative coping tool? If so, what did you do and what happened?

What positive steps did you take to apply self-control to your food/exercise habits, rituals, routines at this session?

ACTIVITY REFLECTION

Journal some thoughts about the meal or snack you selected or the exercise you undertook. Why did you select what you did? Did you have control of your rules, habits, and rituals or did they have control of you?

EMOTION REFLECTION

Journal about the feelings you experienced and how you responded to them. Could you have taken a breath and considered an alternative option? If you did consider and select an alternative, what led you to do that? What allowed you to be more aware of your feelings and responses? If you did not consider an alternative option, what got in the way?

When you complete your last session of Day 20, move on to the Phase Two Reflection.

Phase Two Session Log Sheet

Day 11 - Day 20

Complete the log for this food/exercise session. Place a checkmark next to or circle all that apply.

Date:　　　　　　　　**Day of Week:**　　　　　　　　**Time:**　　　　AM/PM

Reason for the session:　　Meal　　　　Snack　　　　Exercise　　　　Other (Explain)

Meal/Snack location:

　　Dining Table　　　　　Restaurant　　　　　　　　In front of TV/Computer
　　In bed　　　　　　　　Automobile　　　　　　　　Other (Explain)

Beverage Consumed:

　　Soda　　　　　　　　　　Diet soda/seltzer water　　　Tap/bottled water
　　Milk/dairy alternative　　Other (Explain)

Reason for Eating:

　　Nourishment　　　　　　Health　　　　　　　　　　Social Activity/Group Gathering
　　Coping with feelings　　Controlling Emotions　　　Other (Explain)

Exercise Location and Activity:

Who joined you:　　　　　　　　　　**Or Circle:**　　　　Ate Alone/Exercised Alone

Reason for Exercise: (Check or circle the major reasons)

　　Appearance　　　　　　　　　　Fitness
　　Stress/Emotions/Mood　　　　Socializing

Did you count calories eaten or expended?　　Yes　　　No　　　**Why?**

List feelings experienced before/during/after:

How did you respond to those feelings?

Did you think about using an alternative coping tool?   Yes   No

Did you use an alternative coping tool? If so, what did you do and what happened?

What positive steps did you take to apply self-control to your food/exercise habits, rituals, routines at this session?

Activity Reflection

Journal some thoughts about the meal or snack you selected or the exercise you undertook. Why did you select what you did? Did you have control of your rules, habits, and rituals or did they have control of you?

Emotion Reflection

Journal about the feelings you experienced and how you responded to them. Could you have taken a breath and considered an alternative option? If you did consider and select an alternative, what led you to do that? What allowed you to be more aware of your feelings and responses? If you did not consider an alternative option, what got in the way?

When you complete your last session of Day 20, move on to the Phase Two Reflection.

Phase Two Session Log Sheet

Day 11 - Day 20

Complete the log for this food/exercise session. Place a checkmark next to or circle all that apply.

Date: **Day of Week:**   **Time:**   AM/PM

Reason for the session: Meal   Snack   Exercise   Other (Explain)

Meal/Snack location:

Dining Table	Restaurant	In front of TV/Computer
In bed	Automobile	Other (Explain)

Beverage Consumed:

Soda	Diet soda/seltzer water	Tap/bottled water
Milk/dairy alternative	Other (Explain)	

Reason for Eating:

Nourishment	Health	Social Activity/Group Gathering
Coping with feelings	Controlling Emotions	Other (Explain)

Exercise Location and Activity:

Who joined you: **Or Circle:**   Ate Alone/Exercised Alone

Reason for Exercise: (Check or circle the major reasons)

Appearance	Fitness
Stress/Emotions/Mood	Socializing

Did you count calories eaten or expended?   Yes   No   **Why?**

List feelings experienced before/during/after:

How did you respond to those feelings?

Did you think about using an alternative coping tool?   Yes   No

Did you use an alternative coping tool? If so, what did you do and what happened?

What positive steps did you take to apply self-control to your food/exercise habits, rituals, routines at this session?

Activity Reflection

Journal some thoughts about the meal or snack you selected or the exercise you undertook. Why did you select what you did? Did you have control of your rules, habits, and rituals or did they have control of you?

Emotion Reflection

Journal about the feelings you experienced and how you responded to them. Could you have taken a breath and considered an alternative option? If you did consider and select an alternative, what led you to do that? What allowed you to be more aware of your feelings and responses? If you did not consider an alternative option, what got in the way?

When you complete your last session of Day 20, move on to the Phase Two Reflection.

Phase Two Session Log Sheet

Day 11 - Day 20

Complete the log for this food/exercise session. Place a checkmark next to or circle all that apply.

Date: **Day of Week:** **Time:** AM/PM

Reason for the session: Meal Snack Exercise Other (Explain)

Meal/Snack location:

- Dining Table
- In bed
- Restaurant
- Automobile
- In front of TV/Computer
- Other (Explain)

Beverage Consumed:

- Soda
- Milk/dairy alternative
- Diet soda/seltzer water
- Other (Explain)
- Tap/bottled water

Reason for Eating:

- Nourishment
- Coping with feelings
- Health
- Controlling Emotions
- Social Activity/Group Gathering
- Other (Explain)

Exercise Location and Activity:

Who joined you: **Or Circle:** Ate Alone/Exercised Alone

Reason for Exercise: (Check or circle the major reasons)

- Appearance
- Stress/Emotions/Mood
- Fitness
- Socializing

Did you count calories eaten or expended? Yes No **Why?**

List feelings experienced before/during/after:

How did you respond to those feelings?

Did you think about using an alternative coping tool?   Yes   No

Did you use an alternative coping tool? If so, what did you do and what happened?

What positive steps did you take to apply self-control to your food/exercise habits, rituals, routines at this session?

Activity Reflection

Journal some thoughts about the meal or snack you selected or the exercise you undertook. Why did you select what you did? Did you have control of your rules, habits, and rituals or did they have control of you?

Emotion Reflection

Journal about the feelings you experienced and how you responded to them. Could you have taken a breath and considered an alternative option? If you did consider and select an alternative, what led you to do that? What allowed you to be more aware of your feelings and responses? If you did not consider an alternative option, what got in the way?

When you complete your last session of Day 20, move on to the Phase Two Reflection.

Phase Two Session Log Sheet

Day 11 - Day 20

Complete the log for this food/exercise session. Place a checkmark next to or circle all that apply.

Date: **Day of Week:** **Time:** AM/PM

Reason for the session: Meal Snack Exercise Other (Explain)

Meal/Snack location:

    Dining Table Restaurant In front of TV/Computer
    In bed Automobile Other (Explain)

Beverage Consumed:

    Soda Diet soda/seltzer water Tap/bottled water
    Milk/dairy alternative Other (Explain)

Reason for Eating:

    Nourishment Health Social Activity/Group Gathering
    Coping with feelings Controlling Emotions Other (Explain)

Exercise Location and Activity:

Who joined you: **Or Circle:** Ate Alone/Exercised Alone

Reason for Exercise: (Check or circle the major reasons)

    Appearance Fitness
    Stress/Emotions/Mood Socializing

Did you count calories eaten or expended? Yes No **Why?**

List feelings experienced before/during/after:

How did you respond to those feelings?

Did you think about using an alternative coping tool?   Yes   No

Did you use an alternative coping tool? If so, what did you do and what happened?

What positive steps did you take to apply self-control to your food/exercise habits, rituals, routines at this session?

Activity Reflection

Journal some thoughts about the meal or snack you selected or the exercise you undertook. Why did you select what you did? Did you have control of your rules, habits, and rituals or did they have control of you?

Emotion Reflection

Journal about the feelings you experienced and how you responded to them. Could you have taken a breath and considered an alternative option? If you did consider and select an alternative, what led you to do that? What allowed you to be more aware of your feelings and responses? If you did not consider an alternative option, what got in the way?

When you complete your last session of Day 20, move on to the Phase Two Reflection.

Phase Two Session Log Sheet

Day 11 - Day 20

Complete the log for this food/exercise session. Place a checkmark next to or circle all that apply.

Date: **Day of Week:**   **Time:**   AM/PM

Reason for the session: Meal   Snack   Exercise   Other (Explain)

Meal/Snack location:

Dining Table	Restaurant	In front of TV/Computer
In bed	Automobile	Other (Explain)

Beverage Consumed:

Soda	Diet soda/seltzer water	Tap/bottled water
Milk/dairy alternative	Other (Explain)	

Reason for Eating:

Nourishment	Health	Social Activity/Group Gathering
Coping with feelings	Controlling Emotions	Other (Explain)

Exercise Location and Activity:

Who joined you: **Or Circle:**   Ate Alone/Exercised Alone

Reason for Exercise: (Check or circle the major reasons)

Appearance	Fitness
Stress/Emotions/Mood	Socializing

Did you count calories eaten or expended?   Yes   No   **Why?**

List feelings experienced before/during/after:

How did you respond to those feelings?

Did you think about using an alternative coping tool?   Yes   No

Did you use an alternative coping tool? If so, what did you do and what happened?

What positive steps did you take to apply self-control to your food/exercise habits, rituals, routines at this session?

Activity Reflection

Journal some thoughts about the meal or snack you selected or the exercise you undertook. Why did you select what you did? Did you have control of your rules, habits, and rituals or did they have control of you?

Emotion Reflection

Journal about the feelings you experienced and how you responded to them. Could you have taken a breath and considered an alternative option? If you did consider and select an alternative, what led you to do that? What allowed you to be more aware of your feelings and responses? If you did not consider an alternative option, what got in the way?

When you complete your last session of Day 20, move on to the Phase Two Reflection.

Phase Two Session Log Sheet

Day 11 - Day 20

Complete the log for this food/exercise session. Place a checkmark next to or circle all that apply.

Date: **Day of Week:** **Time:** AM/PM

Reason for the session: Meal Snack Exercise Other (Explain)

Meal/Snack location:

Dining Table Restaurant In front of TV/Computer
In bed Automobile Other (Explain)

Beverage Consumed:

Soda Diet soda/seltzer water Tap/bottled water
Milk/dairy alternative Other (Explain)

Reason for Eating:

Nourishment Health Social Activity/Group Gathering
Coping with feelings Controlling Emotions Other (Explain)

Exercise Location and Activity:

Who joined you: **Or Circle:** Ate Alone/Exercised Alone

Reason for Exercise: (Check or circle the major reasons)

Appearance Fitness
Stress/Emotions/Mood Socializing

Did you count calories eaten or expended? Yes No **Why?**

List feelings experienced before/during/after:

How did you respond to those feelings?

Did you think about using an alternative coping tool?   Yes   No

Did you use an alternative coping tool? If so, what did you do and what happened?

What positive steps did you take to apply self-control to your food/exercise habits, rituals, routines at this session?

Activity Reflection

Journal some thoughts about the meal or snack you selected or the exercise you undertook. Why did you select what you did? Did you have control of your rules, habits, and rituals or did they have control of you?

Emotion Reflection

Journal about the feelings you experienced and how you responded to them. Could you have taken a breath and considered an alternative option? If you did consider and select an alternative, what led you to do that? What allowed you to be more aware of your feelings and responses? If you did not consider an alternative option, what got in the way?

When you complete your last session of Day 20, move on to the Phase Two Reflection.

Phase Two Session Log Sheet

Day 11 - Day 20

Complete the log for this food/exercise session. Place a checkmark next to or circle all that apply.

Date: **Day of Week**:   **Time**:   AM/PM

Reason for the session: Meal   Snack   Exercise   Other (Explain)

Meal/Snack location:

    Dining Table   Restaurant   In front of TV/Computer
    In bed   Automobile   Other (Explain)

Beverage Consumed:

    Soda   Diet soda/seltzer water   Tap/bottled water
    Milk/dairy alternative   Other (Explain)

Reason for Eating:

    Nourishment   Health   Social Activity/Group Gathering
    Coping with feelings   Controlling Emotions   Other (Explain)

Exercise Location and Activity:

Who joined you: **Or Circle**:   Ate Alone/Exercised Alone

Reason for Exercise: (Check or circle the major reasons)

    Appearance   Fitness
    Stress/Emotions/Mood   Socializing

Did you count calories eaten or expended?   Yes   No   **Why?**

List feelings experienced before/during/after:

How did you respond to those feelings?

Did you think about using an alternative coping tool?   Yes   No

Did you use an alternative coping tool? If so, what did you do and what happened?

What positive steps did you take to apply self-control to your food/exercise habits, rituals, routines at this session?

ACTIVITY REFLECTION

Journal some thoughts about the meal or snack you selected or the exercise you undertook. Why did you select what you did? Did you have control of your rules, habits, and rituals or did they have control of you?

EMOTION REFLECTION

Journal about the feelings you experienced and how you responded to them. Could you have taken a breath and considered an alternative option? If you did consider and select an alternative, what led you to do that? What allowed you to be more aware of your feelings and responses? If you did not consider an alternative option, what got in the way?

When you complete your last session of Day 20, move on to the Phase Two Reflection.

Phase Two Session Log Sheet

Day 11 - Day 20

Complete the log for this food/exercise session. Place a checkmark next to or circle all that apply.

Date: **Day of Week:**   **Time:**   AM/PM

Reason for the session: Meal   Snack   Exercise   Other (Explain)

Meal/Snack location:

Dining Table	Restaurant	In front of TV/Computer
In bed	Automobile	Other (Explain)

Beverage Consumed:

Soda	Diet soda/seltzer water	Tap/bottled water
Milk/dairy alternative	Other (Explain)	

Reason for Eating:

Nourishment	Health	Social Activity/Group Gathering
Coping with feelings	Controlling Emotions	Other (Explain)

Exercise Location and Activity:

Who joined you: **Or Circle:**   Ate Alone/Exercised Alone

Reason for Exercise: (Check or circle the major reasons)

Appearance	Fitness
Stress/Emotions/Mood	Socializing

Did you count calories eaten or expended?   Yes   No   **Why?**

List feelings experienced before/during/after:

How did you respond to those feelings?

Did you think about using an alternative coping tool?   Yes   No

Did you use an alternative coping tool? If so, what did you do and what happened?

What positive steps did you take to apply self-control to your food/exercise habits, rituals, routines at this session?

ACTIVITY REFLECTION

Journal some thoughts about the meal or snack you selected or the exercise you undertook. Why did you select what you did? Did you have control of your rules, habits, and rituals or did they have control of you?

EMOTION REFLECTION

Journal about the feelings you experienced and how you responded to them. Could you have taken a breath and considered an alternative option? If you did consider and select an alternative, what led you to do that? What allowed you to be more aware of your feelings and responses? If you did not consider an alternative option, what got in the way?

When you complete your last session of Day 20, move on to the Phase Two Reflection.

Phase Two Session Log Sheet

Day 11 - Day 20

Complete the log for this food/exercise session. Place a checkmark next to or circle all that apply.

Date: **Day of Week:**   **Time:**   AM/PM

Reason for the session: Meal   Snack   Exercise   Other (Explain)

Meal/Snack location:

- Dining Table
- In bed
- Restaurant
- Automobile
- In front of TV/Computer
- Other (Explain)

Beverage Consumed:

- Soda
- Milk/dairy alternative
- Diet soda/seltzer water
- Other (Explain)
- Tap/bottled water

Reason for Eating:

- Nourishment
- Coping with feelings
- Health
- Controlling Emotions
- Social Activity/Group Gathering
- Other (Explain)

Exercise Location and Activity:

Who joined you: **Or Circle:**   Ate Alone/Exercised Alone

Reason for Exercise: (Check or circle the major reasons)

- Appearance
- Stress/Emotions/Mood
- Fitness
- Socializing

Did you count calories eaten or expended?   Yes   No   **Why?**

List feelings experienced before/during/after:

How did you respond to those feelings?

Did you think about using an alternative coping tool?   Yes   No

Did you use an alternative coping tool? If so, what did you do and what happened?

What positive steps did you take to apply self-control to your food/exercise habits, rituals, routines at this session?

Activity Reflection

Journal some thoughts about the meal or snack you selected or the exercise you undertook. Why did you select what you did? Did you have control of your rules, habits, and rituals or did they have control of you?

Emotion Reflection

Journal about the feelings you experienced and how you responded to them. Could you have taken a breath and considered an alternative option? If you did consider and select an alternative, what led you to do that? What allowed you to be more aware of your feelings and responses? If you did not consider an alternative option, what got in the way?

When you complete your last session of Day 20, move on to the Phase Two Reflection.

Phase Two Session Log Sheet

Day 11 - Day 20

Complete the log for this food/exercise session. Place a checkmark next to or circle all that apply.

Date: **Day of Week:** **Time:** AM/PM

Reason for the session: Meal   Snack   Exercise   Other (Explain)

Meal/Snack location:

    Dining Table   Restaurant   In front of TV/Computer
    In bed   Automobile   Other (Explain)

Beverage Consumed:

    Soda   Diet soda/seltzer water   Tap/bottled water
    Milk/dairy alternative   Other (Explain)

Reason for Eating:

    Nourishment   Health   Social Activity/Group Gathering
    Coping with feelings   Controlling Emotions   Other (Explain)

Exercise Location and Activity:

Who joined you: **Or Circle:**   Ate Alone/Exercised Alone

Reason for Exercise: (Check or circle the major reasons)

    Appearance   Fitness
    Stress/Emotions/Mood   Socializing

Did you count calories eaten or expended?   Yes   No   **Why?**

List feelings experienced before/during/after:

How did you respond to those feelings?

Did you think about using an alternative coping tool?   Yes   No

Did you use an alternative coping tool? If so, what did you do and what happened?

What positive steps did you take to apply self-control to your food/exercise habits, rituals, routines at this session?

ACTIVITY REFLECTION

Journal some thoughts about the meal or snack you selected or the exercise you undertook. Why did you select what you did? Did you have control of your rules, habits, and rituals or did they have control of you?

EMOTION REFLECTION

Journal about the feelings you experienced and how you responded to them. Could you have taken a breath and considered an alternative option? If you did consider and select an alternative, what led you to do that? What allowed you to be more aware of your feelings and responses? If you did not consider an alternative option, what got in the way?

When you complete your last session of Day 20, move on to the Phase Two Reflection.

Phase Two Session Log Sheet

Day 11 - Day 20

Complete the log for this food/exercise session. Place a checkmark next to or circle all that apply.

Date: **Day of Week:** **Time:** AM/PM

Reason for the session: Meal Snack Exercise Other (Explain)

Meal/Snack location:

    Dining Table Restaurant In front of TV/Computer
    In bed Automobile Other (Explain)

Beverage Consumed:

    Soda Diet soda/seltzer water Tap/bottled water
    Milk/dairy alternative Other (Explain)

Reason for Eating:

    Nourishment Health Social Activity/Group Gathering
    Coping with feelings Controlling Emotions Other (Explain)

Exercise Location and Activity:

Who joined you: **Or Circle:** Ate Alone/Exercised Alone

Reason for Exercise: (Check or circle the major reasons)

    Appearance Fitness
    Stress/Emotions/Mood Socializing

Did you count calories eaten or expended? Yes No **Why?**

List feelings experienced before/during/after:

How did you respond to those feelings?

Did you think about using an alternative coping tool?　　　Yes　　　No

Did you use an alternative coping tool? If so, what did you do and what happened?

What positive steps did you take to apply self-control to your food/exercise habits, rituals, routines at this session?

Activity Reflection

Journal some thoughts about the meal or snack you selected or the exercise you undertook. Why did you select what you did? Did you have control of your rules, habits, and rituals or did they have control of you?

Emotion Reflection

Journal about the feelings you experienced and how you responded to them. Could you have taken a breath and considered an alternative option? If you did consider and select an alternative, what led you to do that? What allowed you to be more aware of your feelings and responses? If you did not consider an alternative option, what got in the way?

When you complete your last session of Day 20, move on to the Phase Two Reflection.

Phase Two Session Log Sheet

Day 11 - Day 20

Complete the log for this food/exercise session. Place a checkmark next to or circle all that apply.

Date: **Day of Week:**   **Time:**   AM/PM

Reason for the session: Meal   Snack   Exercise   Other (Explain)

Meal/Snack location:

     Dining Table   Restaurant   In front of TV/Computer
     In bed   Automobile   Other (Explain)

Beverage Consumed:

     Soda   Diet soda/seltzer water   Tap/bottled water
     Milk/dairy alternative   Other (Explain)

Reason for Eating:

     Nourishment   Health   Social Activity/Group Gathering
     Coping with feelings   Controlling Emotions   Other (Explain)

Exercise Location and Activity:

Who joined you: **Or Circle:**   Ate Alone/Exercised Alone

Reason for Exercise: (Check or circle the major reasons)

     Appearance   Fitness
     Stress/Emotions/Mood   Socializing

Did you count calories eaten or expended?   Yes   No   **Why?**

List feelings experienced before/during/after:

How did you respond to those feelings?

Did you think about using an alternative coping tool?   Yes   No

Did you use an alternative coping tool? If so, what did you do and what happened?

What positive steps did you take to apply self-control to your food/exercise habits, rituals, routines at this session?

ACTIVITY REFLECTION

Journal some thoughts about the meal or snack you selected or the exercise you undertook. Why did you select what you did? Did you have control of your rules, habits, and rituals or did they have control of you?

EMOTION REFLECTION

Journal about the feelings you experienced and how you responded to them. Could you have taken a breath and considered an alternative option? If you did consider and select an alternative, what led you to do that? What allowed you to be more aware of your feelings and responses? If you did not consider an alternative option, what got in the way?

When you complete your last session of Day 20, move on to the Phase Two Reflection.

Phase Two Session Log Sheet

Day 11 – Day 20

Complete the log for this food/exercise session. Place a checkmark next to or circle all that apply.

Date: **Day of Week:**   **Time:**   AM/PM

Reason for the session: Meal   Snack   Exercise   Other (Explain)

Meal/Snack location:

    Dining Table   Restaurant   In front of TV/Computer
    In bed   Automobile   Other (Explain)

Beverage Consumed:

    Soda   Diet soda/seltzer water   Tap/bottled water
    Milk/dairy alternative   Other (Explain)

Reason for Eating:

    Nourishment   Health   Social Activity/Group Gathering
    Coping with feelings   Controlling Emotions   Other (Explain)

Exercise Location and Activity:

Who joined you: **Or Circle:**   Ate Alone/Exercised Alone

Reason for Exercise: (Check or circle the major reasons)

    Appearance   Fitness
    Stress/Emotions/Mood   Socializing

Did you count calories eaten or expended?   Yes   No   **Why?**

List feelings experienced before/during/after:

How did you respond to those feelings?

Did you think about using an alternative coping tool?   Yes   No

Did you use an alternative coping tool? If so, what did you do and what happened?

What positive steps did you take to apply self-control to your food/exercise habits, rituals, routines at this session?

Activity Reflection

Journal some thoughts about the meal or snack you selected or the exercise you undertook. Why did you select what you did? Did you have control of your rules, habits, and rituals or did they have control of you?

Emotion Reflection

Journal about the feelings you experienced and how you responded to them. Could you have taken a breath and considered an alternative option? If you did consider and select an alternative, what led you to do that? What allowed you to be more aware of your feelings and responses? If you did not consider an alternative option, what got in the way?

When you complete your last session of Day 20, move on to the Phase Two Reflection.

Phase Two Session Log Sheet

Day 11 - Day 20

Complete the log for this food/exercise session. Place a checkmark next to or circle all that apply.

Date:　　　　　　　　**Day of Week**:　　　　　　　　**Time**:　　　　　AM/PM

Reason for the session:　　Meal　　　　Snack　　　　Exercise　　　　Other (Explain)

Meal/Snack location:

　　Dining Table　　　　　Restaurant　　　　　　　　In front of TV/Computer
　　In bed　　　　　　　　Automobile　　　　　　　　Other (Explain)

Beverage Consumed:

　　Soda　　　　　　　　　Diet soda/seltzer water　　　Tap/bottled water
　　Milk/dairy alternative　Other (Explain)

Reason for Eating:

　　Nourishment　　　　　Health　　　　　　　　　　Social Activity/Group Gathering
　　Coping with feelings　Controlling Emotions　　　Other (Explain)

Exercise Location and Activity:

Who joined you:　　　　　　　　　　　**Or Circle**:　　　　Ate Alone/Exercised Alone

Reason for Exercise: (Check or circle the major reasons)

　　Appearance　　　　　　　　　Fitness
　　Stress/Emotions/Mood　　　　Socializing

Did you count calories eaten or expended?　　Yes　　　No　　　**Why?**

List feelings experienced before/during/after:

How did you respond to those feelings?

Did you think about using an alternative coping tool?   Yes   No

Did you use an alternative coping tool? If so, what did you do and what happened?

What positive steps did you take to apply self-control to your food/exercise habits, rituals, routines at this session?

Activity Reflection

Journal some thoughts about the meal or snack you selected or the exercise you undertook. Why did you select what you did? Did you have control of your rules, habits, and rituals or did they have control of you?

Emotion Reflection

Journal about the feelings you experienced and how you responded to them. Could you have taken a breath and considered an alternative option? If you did consider and select an alternative, what led you to do that? What allowed you to be more aware of your feelings and responses? If you did not consider an alternative option, what got in the way?

When you complete your last session of Day 20, move on to the Phase Two Reflection.

Phase Two Session Log Sheet

Day 11 - Day 20

Complete the log for this food/exercise session. Place a checkmark next to or circle all that apply.

Date:　　　　　　　　　**Day of Week:**　　　　　　　**Time:**　　　　　AM/PM

Reason for the session:　　Meal　　　　Snack　　　　Exercise　　　　Other (Explain)

Meal/Snack location:

　　Dining Table　　　　　Restaurant　　　　　　　　In front of TV/Computer
　　In bed　　　　　　　　Automobile　　　　　　　　Other (Explain)

Beverage Consumed:

　　Soda　　　　　　　　　　Diet soda/seltzer water　　Tap/bottled water
　　Milk/dairy alternative　　Other (Explain)

Reason for Eating:

　　Nourishment　　　　　　Health　　　　　　　　　　Social Activity/Group Gathering
　　Coping with feelings　　Controlling Emotions　　　Other (Explain)

Exercise Location and Activity:

Who joined you:　　　　　　　　　　**Or Circle:**　　　　Ate Alone/Exercised Alone

Reason for Exercise: (Check or circle the major reasons)

　　Appearance　　　　　　　　　Fitness
　　Stress/Emotions/Mood　　　　Socializing

Did you count calories eaten or expended?　　Yes　　　No　　　**Why?**

List feelings experienced before/during/after:

How did you respond to those feelings?

Did you think about using an alternative coping tool?   Yes   No

Did you use an alternative coping tool? If so, what did you do and what happened?

What positive steps did you take to apply self-control to your food/exercise habits, rituals, routines at this session?

ACTIVITY REFLECTION

Journal some thoughts about the meal or snack you selected or the exercise you undertook. Why did you select what you did? Did you have control of your rules, habits, and rituals or did they have control of you?

EMOTION REFLECTION

Journal about the feelings you experienced and how you responded to them. Could you have taken a breath and considered an alternative option? If you did consider and select an alternative, what led you to do that? What allowed you to be more aware of your feelings and responses? If you did not consider an alternative option, what got in the way?

When you complete your last session of Day 20, move on to the Phase Two Reflection.

Phase Two Session Log Sheet

Day 11 - Day 20

Complete the log for this food/exercise session. Place a checkmark next to or circle all that apply.

Date:　　　　　　　　**Day of Week:**　　　　　　　**Time:**　　　　　　AM/PM

Reason for the session:　　Meal　　　　Snack　　　　Exercise　　　　Other (Explain)

Meal/Snack location:

　　Dining Table　　　　　　Restaurant　　　　　　　　In front of TV/Computer
　　In bed　　　　　　　　　Automobile　　　　　　　　Other (Explain)

Beverage Consumed:

　　Soda　　　　　　　　　　Diet soda/seltzer water　　　Tap/bottled water
　　Milk/dairy alternative　　Other (Explain)

Reason for Eating:

　　Nourishment　　　　　　Health　　　　　　　　　　Social Activity/Group Gathering
　　Coping with feelings　　Controlling Emotions　　　　Other (Explain)

Exercise Location and Activity:

Who joined you:　　　　　　　　　　　**Or Circle:**　　　　Ate Alone/Exercised Alone

Reason for Exercise: (Check or circle the major reasons)

　　Appearance　　　　　　　　　　　Fitness
　　Stress/Emotions/Mood　　　　　　Socializing

Did you count calories eaten or expended?　　Yes　　　No　　　**Why?**

List feelings experienced before/during/after:

How did you respond to those feelings?

Did you think about using an alternative coping tool?   Yes   No

Did you use an alternative coping tool? If so, what did you do and what happened?

What positive steps did you take to apply self-control to your food/exercise habits, rituals, routines at this session?

Activity Reflection

Journal some thoughts about the meal or snack you selected or the exercise you undertook. Why did you select what you did? Did you have control of your rules, habits, and rituals or did they have control of you?

Emotion Reflection

Journal about the feelings you experienced and how you responded to them. Could you have taken a breath and considered an alternative option? If you did consider and select an alternative, what led you to do that? What allowed you to be more aware of your feelings and responses? If you did not consider an alternative option, what got in the way?

When you complete your last session of Day 20, move on to the Phase Two Reflection.

Phase Two Session Log Sheet

Day 11 - Day 20

Complete the log for this food/exercise session. Place a checkmark next to or circle all that apply.

Date: **Day of Week:**   **Time:**   AM/PM

Reason for the session: Meal   Snack   Exercise   Other (Explain)

Meal/Snack location:

Dining Table	Restaurant	In front of TV/Computer
In bed	Automobile	Other (Explain)

Beverage Consumed:

Soda	Diet soda/seltzer water	Tap/bottled water
Milk/dairy alternative	Other (Explain)	

Reason for Eating:

Nourishment	Health	Social Activity/Group Gathering
Coping with feelings	Controlling Emotions	Other (Explain)

Exercise Location and Activity:

Who joined you: **Or Circle:**   Ate Alone/Exercised Alone

Reason for Exercise: (Check or circle the major reasons)

Appearance	Fitness
Stress/Emotions/Mood	Socializing

Did you count calories eaten or expended?   Yes   No   **Why?**

List feelings experienced before/during/after:

How did you respond to those feelings?

Did you think about using an alternative coping tool?   Yes   No

Did you use an alternative coping tool? If so, what did you do and what happened?

What positive steps did you take to apply self-control to your food/exercise habits, rituals, routines at this session?

Activity Reflection

Journal some thoughts about the meal or snack you selected or the exercise you undertook. Why did you select what you did? Did you have control of your rules, habits, and rituals or did they have control of you?

Emotion Reflection

Journal about the feelings you experienced and how you responded to them. Could you have taken a breath and considered an alternative option? If you did consider and select an alternative, what led you to do that? What allowed you to be more aware of your feelings and responses? If you did not consider an alternative option, what got in the way?

When you complete your last session of Day 20, move on to the Phase Two Reflection.

Phase Two Session Log Sheet

Day 11 - Day 20

Complete the log for this food/exercise session. Place a checkmark next to or circle all that apply.

Date:　　　　　　　　**Day of Week:**　　　　　　　　**Time:**　　　　　AM/PM

Reason for the session:　　Meal　　　　Snack　　　　Exercise　　　　Other (Explain)

Meal/Snack location:

　　Dining Table　　　　　　Restaurant　　　　　　　　In front of TV/Computer
　　In bed　　　　　　　　　Automobile　　　　　　　　Other (Explain)

Beverage Consumed:

　　Soda　　　　　　　　　　Diet soda/seltzer water　　　Tap/bottled water
　　Milk/dairy alternative　　Other (Explain)

Reason for Eating:

　　Nourishment　　　　　　Health　　　　　　　　　　Social Activity/Group Gathering
　　Coping with feelings　　Controlling Emotions　　　Other (Explain)

Exercise Location and Activity:

Who joined you:　　　　　　　　　　**Or Circle:**　　　　　Ate Alone/Exercised Alone

Reason for Exercise: (Check or circle the major reasons)

　　Appearance　　　　　　　　　　　　Fitness
　　Stress/Emotions/Mood　　　　　　Socializing

Did you count calories eaten or expended?　　Yes　　No　　**Why?**

List feelings experienced before/during/after:

How did you respond to those feelings?

Did you think about using an alternative coping tool?   Yes   No

Did you use an alternative coping tool? If so, what did you do and what happened?

What positive steps did you take to apply self-control to your food/exercise habits, rituals, routines at this session?

Activity Reflection

Journal some thoughts about the meal or snack you selected or the exercise you undertook. Why did you select what you did? Did you have control of your rules, habits, and rituals or did they have control of you?

Emotion Reflection

Journal about the feelings you experienced and how you responded to them. Could you have taken a breath and considered an alternative option? If you did consider and select an alternative, what led you to do that? What allowed you to be more aware of your feelings and responses? If you did not consider an alternative option, what got in the way?

When you complete your last session of Day 20, move on to the Phase Two Reflection.

**If you need more pages for Phase Two, you will find
an additional form to copy in the Appendix**

Phase Two Reflection

Congratulations on completing the second phase of your mindfulness journey! Now it is time to look back at where you have been over the last ten days. Look for small steps you took to apply self-control that managed your rules, habits, and rituals through conscience thought and positive alternatives. Be honest regarding the places you didn't apply self-control and own the reasons why.

Take a few moments to honestly answer the following questions.

On average, how many times did you eat a meal or snack each day? What was the average time interval between them?

Was this different from Phase One? How was it different? What led to the change? If it isn't any different, what prevented change?

On average, how many times did you exercise each day? What was the average duration of the session?

Was this different from Phase One? How is it different? What led to the change? If it isn't any different, what prevented change?

Over the past ten days, did you see any changes in your reason for your sessions? If so, what led to the change? If not, what prevented a change?

Who joined you most often or did you participate alone most often? How do you feel about that?

Did you find you experienced different feelings before, during, or after your sessions over the last ten days compared to Phase One? If so, what facilitated those changes? If not, what allowed them to persist?

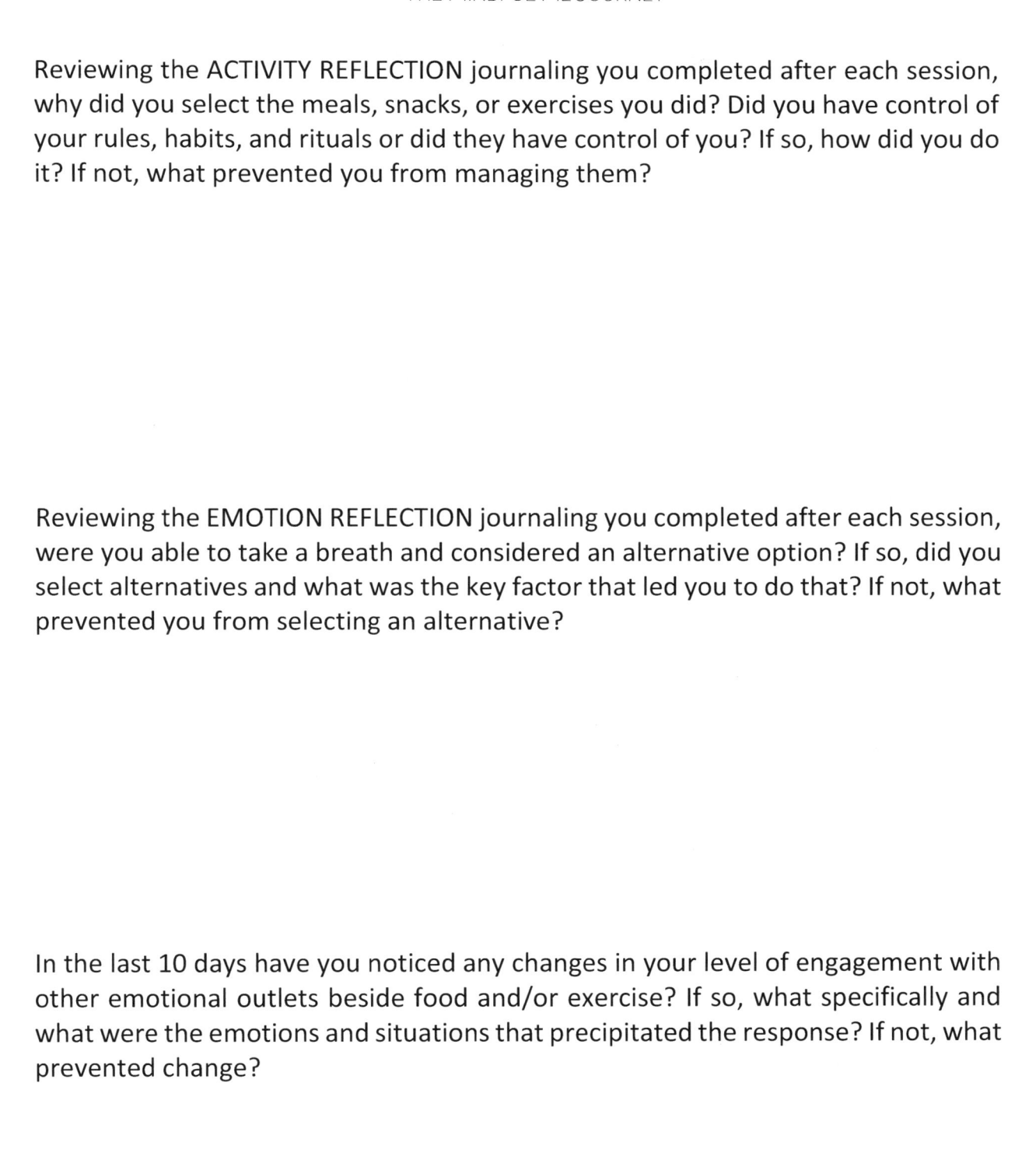

Reviewing the ACTIVITY REFLECTION journaling you completed after each session, why did you select the meals, snacks, or exercises you did? Did you have control of your rules, habits, and rituals or did they have control of you? If so, how did you do it? If not, what prevented you from managing them?

Reviewing the EMOTION REFLECTION journaling you completed after each session, were you able to take a breath and considered an alternative option? If so, did you select alternatives and what was the key factor that led you to do that? If not, what prevented you from selecting an alternative?

In the last 10 days have you noticed any changes in your level of engagement with other emotional outlets beside food and/or exercise? If so, what specifically and what were the emotions and situations that precipitated the response? If not, what prevented change?

Phase Three

Beginning to Build an Individualized Plan

Hopefully, after completing the last two phases of your journey, you are becoming more aware of the choices you are making as you respond to the feelings and emotions you are experiencing. In this next phase you will begin to make positive mindful decisions related to food and exercise. You want to begin moving away from manipulation at the expense of your body and health toward loving choices that care for your body and health.

Since we are each unique and an experiment of one, there is no one size fits all food or fitness plan to facilitate good health. You *can* build an individual plan that helps you restore and maintain good health. The goal is to select healthy and nutrient rich meals, snacks, and beverages that nourish the body. You want to be physically active and engaging in regular cardiovascular and weight-bearing activities that maintain good health, limit disease, and assist in the management of medical conditions that may exist.

At the same time, it is important to recognize our hang ups and barriers so we can put plans in place that help us take small but strategic steps forward. A guardrail on the roadway is intended to prevent a motorist from going off the road. They are there to make the road safer and to lessen the severity of a crash. In the same way, we can apply food and exercise guardrails that help us stay on the road to better health and prevent crashing into old rules, habits, and rituals that seek to derail us.

Here are a few examples of what I mean. If you have been a restrictor of food, I would bet the idea of eating directly out of the bag is very terrifying. The reason for that would be that you are used to controlling your portion sizes and knowing exactly how many calories you consume. A strategic guardrail for you might be to eat right out of the bag. Reversely, if you are a binge eater, eating out of the bag and not limiting your portion size is a trigger for you. A strategic guardrail for you might be to take a portion out of the bag, put it on a plate, and sit at a table to eat instead of in front of a TV, computer, or in your car. Both of these approaches are mindful choices made to take you forward from where you are, toward where you need to go at your pace. Both of these actions will be a step that can be a struggle and that will bring a variety of thoughts, feelings, and emotions which you would have to confront. However, this is the hard but important step you need so you can work through and break the chains that hold you to diets and disorder.

The same is true for exercise. The American Heart Association recommends regular moderate to vigorous intensity aerobic activity spread throughout the week for good health. Are you someone who exercises with a smartwatch that tells you exactly how many calories you have burned and how many minutes in your week was moderate or vigorous activity? Exercising without your smartwatch and having no idea of calories expended or how much time was spent in various exercise levels could be panic inducing. However, it could be just the guardrail you need to help you break the chains and begin recovery. Reversely, are you someone that isn't regularly active or only tracks steps and has trouble meeting 5,000 steps a day? You may benefit from paying more attention to the amount of activity you get and at what level to help you take steps forward in activity for health. Both of these actions will be steps that can be a struggle and can bring a variety of thoughts, feelings, and emotions which you will have to confront. But these are the small steps forward that lead you toward better health.

Here are some guidelines and guardrails to help you become more mindful during these next ten days.

- Put away your focus on the number of calories related to food. Begin to focus instead on the nutrition of food and how your selections will nourish your body. Begin to focus on the ingredients, manner of preparation, and how they influence your senses. The same is true for the calories expended in exercise. Begin to focus on how your body is responding to the activity. Take note of the level of your heart rate, the rate of your breathing, and the fatigue of your muscles. Take notice of the sights, sounds, and smells around you as you eat or exercise as well as what you are thinking about or focusing on.
- Be mindful of your previous areas of abuse to your body such as restriction, over-exercise, over-consumption, binging, purging, or laxative abuse and put guardrails up that will limit triggers or will help you change a behavior in its tracks.

- Build in new activities related to food and exercise selection that will help you take a step beyond your past areas of abuse or control. Introduce a new food, cook in a healthier way, or apply a new guardrail to help you stay on task and moving forward.
- Remember that hunger describes the escalating, physiological sensation you experience when your body needs food. It is normal and it not to be ignored. It is the innate signal that your body needs something. Whether that is energy, protein, or water is for you to discover. Most people who eat a balanced diet with adequate calories experience hunger cues beginning about four hours after the last meal and they will escalate after about five hours.
- A physical feeling of fullness is known as satiety. It can take up to 20 minutes for your brain to receive the signal that your stomach is full and to return the "stop eating" signal. Take your time eating and be mindful about how you are physically feeling while you eat versus focusing on emotional feelings as you eat. Take note of how you feel physically after you eat related to the choices that you made.
- Making mindful choices requires three skills:
    - The ability to recognize innate hunger and satiety signals.
    - The ability to distinguish between hunger, appetite (which include your preferences, habits, and tastes), and your impulse.
    - The ability to stay grounded in yourself so that you are making the decisions instead of your hunger, appetite, impulses, or diet rules making them.

During the next ten days you will complete a session log for *each* food or exercise related activity you undertake just as you did over the last twenty days. Ideally you will use a *new entry* for each session. However, if you do not have the time to commit to that level of discovery, doing one entry at the end of the day that captures the highlights is also an option. If you run out of session journal entry space before your last session on day 30, please go to the appendix section of the journal and make additional copies. If you get to your last session of day 30 and you aren't at the end of the provided Phase Three journaling pages, move on to the Phase Three Reflection activity. Once you have completed your last session on day 30, take some time to complete the *Phase Three Reflection* questions. Be sure to allow time to reflect and journal after *each* session as well as at the end of day 30.

Phase Three Session Log Sheet

Day 21 - Day 30

Complete the log for this food/exercise session. Place a checkmark next to or circle all that apply.

Date:　　　　　　　　**Day of Week:**　　　　　　　　**Time:**　　　　　　AM/PM

Reason for the session:　　Meal　　　　Snack　　　　Exercise　　　　Other (Explain)

Meal Components:　　Protein　　Fruit　　Whole grain　　Vegetable　　Healthy Fat

Method of Preparation:

Baked	Broiled	Sautéed	Grilled	Boiled
Fried	Roasted	Steamed	Stir-fry	Stewed
Fresh/raw	Frozen	Canned	Processed/packaged	
Prepared by others	Other (Explain)			

Beverage Consumed:

Soda	Diet soda/seltzer water	Tap/bottled water
Milk/dairy alternative	Other (Explain)	

Exercise Location and Activity:

Level of Activity:　　　　Easy　　　　Moderate　　　　Vigorous　　　　Highly Vigorous

Who joined you:　　　　　　　　**Or Circle:**　　　　Ate Alone/Exercised Alone

Feelings experienced before/during/after and how you responded to those feelings? Were they expressed in the session? If so, how and if not, why not?

What positive step did you take or guardrail did you apply during this session? Did it go as planned? Would you do anything differently next time?

Activity Reflection

Journal some thoughts about the meal or snack you selected or the exercise you undertook. How did the meal/snack look, smell, and taste? What did you notice going on around you as you exercised? How were you in control of this session and how did this session control you?

Emotion Reflection

Journal about the feelings you experienced and how you responded to them. Was this session a reflection of feelings and emotions? List some positive self-talk responses you can offer to your internal critic to combat the lies you hear in your head.

When you complete your last session of Day 30, move on to the Phase Three Reflection.

Phase Three Session Log Sheet

Day 21 - Day 30

Complete the log for this food/exercise session. Place a checkmark next to or circle all that apply.

Date: **Day of Week:** **Time:** AM/PM

Reason for the session: Meal Snack Exercise Other (Explain)

Meal Components: Protein Fruit Whole grain Vegetable Healthy Fat

Method of Preparation:

Baked	Broiled	Sautéed	Grilled	Boiled
Fried	Roasted	Steamed	Stir-fry	Stewed
Fresh/raw	Frozen	Canned	Processed/packaged	
Prepared by others	Other (Explain)			

Beverage Consumed:

Soda Diet soda/seltzer water Tap/bottled water
Milk/dairy alternative Other (Explain)

Exercise Location and Activity:

Level of Activity: Easy Moderate Vigorous Highly Vigorous

Who joined you: **Or Circle:** Ate Alone/Exercised Alone

Feelings experienced before/during/after and how you responded to those feelings? Were they expressed in the session? If so, how and if not, why not?

What positive step did you take or guardrail did you apply during this session? Did it go as planned? Would you do anything differently next time?

ACTIVITY REFLECTION

Journal some thoughts about the meal or snack you selected or the exercise you undertook. How did the meal/snack look, smell, and taste? What did you notice going on around you as you exercised? How were you in control of this session and how did this session control you?

EMOTION REFLECTION

Journal about the feelings you experienced and how you responded to them. Was this session a reflection of feelings and emotions? List some positive self-talk responses you can offer to your internal critic to combat the lies you hear in your head.

When you complete your last session of Day 30, move on to the Phase Three Reflection.

Phase Three Session Log Sheet

Day 21 - Day 30

Complete the log for this food/exercise session. Place a checkmark next to or circle all that apply.

Date: **Day of Week:**   **Time:**   AM/PM

Reason for the session: Meal   Snack   Exercise   Other (Explain)

Meal Components: Protein   Fruit   Whole grain   Vegetable   Healthy Fat

Method of Preparation:

Baked	Broiled	Sautéed	Grilled	Boiled
Fried	Roasted	Steamed	Stir-fry	Stewed
Fresh/raw	Frozen	Canned	Processed/packaged	
Prepared by others	Other (Explain)			

Beverage Consumed:

Soda   Diet soda/seltzer water   Tap/bottled water
Milk/dairy alternative   Other (Explain)

Exercise Location and Activity:

Level of Activity: Easy   Moderate   Vigorous   Highly Vigorous

Who joined you: **Or Circle:**   Ate Alone/Exercised Alone

Feelings experienced before/during/after and how you responded to those feelings? Were they expressed in the session? If so, how and if not, why not?

What positive step did you take or guardrail did you apply during this session? Did it go as planned? Would you do anything differently next time?

Activity Reflection

Journal some thoughts about the meal or snack you selected or the exercise you undertook. How did the meal/snack look, smell, and taste? What did you notice going on around you as you exercised? How were you in control of this session and how did this session control you?

Emotion Reflection

Journal about the feelings you experienced and how you responded to them. Was this session a reflection of feelings and emotions? List some positive self-talk responses you can offer to your internal critic to combat the lies you hear in your head.

When you complete your last session of Day 30, move on to the Phase Three Reflection.

Phase Three Session Log Sheet

Day 21 - Day 30

Complete the log for this food/exercise session. Place a checkmark next to or circle all that apply.

Date: **Day of Week:**   **Time:**   AM/PM

Reason for the session: Meal   Snack   Exercise   Other (Explain)

Meal Components: Protein   Fruit   Whole grain   Vegetable   Healthy Fat

Method of Preparation:

Baked	Broiled	Sautéed	Grilled	Boiled
Fried	Roasted	Steamed	Stir-fry	Stewed
Fresh/raw	Frozen	Canned	Processed/packaged	
Prepared by others	Other (Explain)			

Beverage Consumed:

Soda	Diet soda/seltzer water	Tap/bottled water
Milk/dairy alternative	Other (Explain)	

Exercise Location and Activity:

Level of Activity: Easy   Moderate   Vigorous   Highly Vigorous

Who joined you: **Or Circle:**   Ate Alone/Exercised Alone

Feelings experienced before/during/after and how you responded to those feelings? Were they expressed in the session? If so, how and if not, why not?

What positive step did you take or guardrail did you apply during this session? Did it go as planned? Would you do anything differently next time?

ACTIVITY REFLECTION

Journal some thoughts about the meal or snack you selected or the exercise you undertook. How did the meal/snack look, smell, and taste? What did you notice going on around you as you exercised? How were you in control of this session and how did this session control you?

EMOTION REFLECTION

Journal about the feelings you experienced and how you responded to them. Was this session a reflection of feelings and emotions? List some positive self-talk responses you can offer to your internal critic to combat the lies you hear in your head.

When you complete your last session of Day 30, move on to the Phase Three Reflection.

Phase Three Session Log Sheet

Day 21 - Day 30

Complete the log for this food/exercise session. Place a checkmark next to or circle all that apply.

Date: **Day of Week:**   **Time:**   AM/PM

Reason for the session: Meal   Snack   Exercise   Other (Explain)

Meal Components: Protein   Fruit   Whole grain   Vegetable   Healthy Fat

Method of Preparation:

Baked	Broiled	Sautéed	Grilled	Boiled
Fried	Roasted	Steamed	Stir-fry	Stewed
Fresh/raw	Frozen	Canned	Processed/packaged	
Prepared by others	Other (Explain)			

Beverage Consumed:

Soda   Diet soda/seltzer water   Tap/bottled water
Milk/dairy alternative   Other (Explain)

Exercise Location and Activity:

Level of Activity: Easy   Moderate   Vigorous   Highly Vigorous

Who joined you: **Or Circle:**   Ate Alone/Exercised Alone

Feelings experienced before/during/after and how you responded to those feelings? Were they expressed in the session? If so, how and if not, why not?

What positive step did you take or guardrail did you apply during this session? Did it go as planned? Would you do anything differently next time?

ACTIVITY REFLECTION

Journal some thoughts about the meal or snack you selected or the exercise you undertook. How did the meal/snack look, smell, and taste? What did you notice going on around you as you exercised? How were you in control of this session and how did this session control you?

EMOTION REFLECTION

Journal about the feelings you experienced and how you responded to them. Was this session a reflection of feelings and emotions? List some positive self-talk responses you can offer to your internal critic to combat the lies you hear in your head.

When you complete your last session of Day 30, move on to the Phase Three Reflection.

Phase Three Session Log Sheet

Day 21 - Day 30

Complete the log for this food/exercise session. Place a checkmark next to or circle all that apply.

Date:　　　　　　　　**Day of Week:**　　　　　　　**Time:**　　　　　AM/PM

Reason for the session:　　Meal　　　　Snack　　　　Exercise　　　　Other (Explain)

Meal Components:　　Protein　　Fruit　　Whole grain　　Vegetable　　Healthy Fat

Method of Preparation:

Baked	Broiled	Sautéed	Grilled	Boiled
Fried	Roasted	Steamed	Stir-fry	Stewed
Fresh/raw	Frozen	Canned	Processed/packaged	
Prepared by others	Other (Explain)			

Beverage Consumed:

Soda　　　　　　　　　Diet soda/seltzer water　　　　Tap/bottled water
Milk/dairy alternative　　Other (Explain)

Exercise Location and Activity:

Level of Activity:　　　Easy　　　　Moderate　　　　Vigorous　　　　Highly Vigorous

Who joined you:　　　　　　　　　**Or Circle:**　　　Ate Alone/Exercised Alone

Feelings experienced before/during/after and how you responded to those feelings? Were they expressed in the session? If so, how and if not, why not?

What positive step did you take or guardrail did you apply during this session? Did it go as planned? Would you do anything differently next time?

Activity Reflection

Journal some thoughts about the meal or snack you selected or the exercise you undertook. How did the meal/snack look, smell, and taste? What did you notice going on around you as you exercised? How were you in control of this session and how did this session control you?

Emotion Reflection

Journal about the feelings you experienced and how you responded to them. Was this session a reflection of feelings and emotions? List some positive self-talk responses you can offer to your internal critic to combat the lies you hear in your head.

When you complete your last session of Day 30, move on to the Phase Three Reflection.

Phase Three Session Log Sheet

Day 21 - Day 30

Complete the log for this food/exercise session. Place a checkmark next to or circle all that apply.

Date: **Day of Week:**   **Time:**   AM/PM

Reason for the session: Meal   Snack   Exercise   Other (Explain)

Meal Components: Protein   Fruit   Whole grain   Vegetable   Healthy Fat

Method of Preparation:

Baked	Broiled	Sautéed	Grilled	Boiled
Fried	Roasted	Steamed	Stir-fry	Stewed
Fresh/raw	Frozen	Canned	Processed/packaged	
Prepared by others	Other (Explain)			

Beverage Consumed:

Soda   Diet soda/seltzer water   Tap/bottled water
Milk/dairy alternative   Other (Explain)

Exercise Location and Activity:

Level of Activity: Easy   Moderate   Vigorous   Highly Vigorous

Who joined you: **Or Circle:**   Ate Alone/Exercised Alone

Feelings experienced before/during/after and how you responded to those feelings? Were they expressed in the session? If so, how and if not, why not?

What positive step did you take or guardrail did you apply during this session? Did it go as planned? Would you do anything differently next time?

Activity Reflection

Journal some thoughts about the meal or snack you selected or the exercise you undertook. How did the meal/snack look, smell, and taste? What did you notice going on around you as you exercised? How were you in control of this session and how did this session control you?

Emotion Reflection

Journal about the feelings you experienced and how you responded to them. Was this session a reflection of feelings and emotions? List some positive self-talk responses you can offer to your internal critic to combat the lies you hear in your head.

When you complete your last session of Day 30, move on to the Phase Three Reflection.

Phase Three Session Log Sheet

Day 21 - Day 30

Complete the log for this food/exercise session. Place a checkmark next to or circle all that apply.

Date: **Day of Week:** **Time:** AM/PM

Reason for the session: Meal Snack Exercise Other (Explain)

Meal Components: Protein Fruit Whole grain Vegetable Healthy Fat

Method of Preparation:

Baked	Broiled	Sautéed	Grilled	Boiled
Fried	Roasted	Steamed	Stir-fry	Stewed
Fresh/raw	Frozen	Canned	Processed/packaged	
Prepared by others	Other (Explain)			

Beverage Consumed:

Soda Diet soda/seltzer water Tap/bottled water
Milk/dairy alternative Other (Explain)

Exercise Location and Activity:

Level of Activity: Easy Moderate Vigorous Highly Vigorous

Who joined you: **Or Circle:** Ate Alone/Exercised Alone

Feelings experienced before/during/after and how you responded to those feelings? Were they expressed in the session? If so, how and if not, why not?

What positive step did you take or guardrail did you apply during this session? Did it go as planned? Would you do anything differently next time?

Activity Reflection

Journal some thoughts about the meal or snack you selected or the exercise you undertook. How did the meal/snack look, smell, and taste? What did you notice going on around you as you exercised? How were you in control of this session and how did this session control you?

Emotion Reflection

Journal about the feelings you experienced and how you responded to them. Was this session a reflection of feelings and emotions? List some positive self-talk responses you can offer to your internal critic to combat the lies you hear in your head.

When you complete your last session of Day 30, move on to the Phase Three Reflection.

Phase Three Session Log Sheet

Day 21 - Day 30

Complete the log for this food/exercise session. Place a checkmark next to or circle all that apply.

Date: **Day of Week**:   **Time**:   AM/PM

Reason for the session: Meal   Snack   Exercise   Other (Explain)

Meal Components: Protein   Fruit   Whole grain   Vegetable   Healthy Fat

Method of Preparation:

Baked	Broiled	Sautéed	Grilled	Boiled
Fried	Roasted	Steamed	Stir-fry	Stewed
Fresh/raw	Frozen	Canned	Processed/packaged	
Prepared by others	Other (Explain)			

Beverage Consumed:

Soda	Diet soda/seltzer water	Tap/bottled water
Milk/dairy alternative	Other (Explain)	

Exercise Location and Activity:

Level of Activity: Easy   Moderate   Vigorous   Highly Vigorous

Who joined you: **Or Circle:**   Ate Alone/Exercised Alone

Feelings experienced before/during/after and how you responded to those feelings? Were they expressed in the session? If so, how and if not, why not?

What positive step did you take or guardrail did you apply during this session? Did it go as planned? Would you do anything differently next time?

ACTIVITY REFLECTION

Journal some thoughts about the meal or snack you selected or the exercise you undertook. How did the meal/snack look, smell, and taste? What did you notice going on around you as you exercised? How were you in control of this session and how did this session control you?

EMOTION REFLECTION

Journal about the feelings you experienced and how you responded to them. Was this session a reflection of feelings and emotions? List some positive self-talk responses you can offer to your internal critic to combat the lies you hear in your head.

When you complete your last session of Day 30, move on to the Phase Three Reflection.

Phase Three Session Log Sheet

Day 21 - Day 30

Complete the log for this food/exercise session. Place a checkmark next to or circle all that apply.

Date: **Day of Week:**   **Time:**   AM/PM

Reason for the session: Meal   Snack   Exercise   Other (Explain)

Meal Components: Protein   Fruit   Whole grain   Vegetable   Healthy Fat

Method of Preparation:

Baked	Broiled	Sautéed	Grilled	Boiled
Fried	Roasted	Steamed	Stir-fry	Stewed
Fresh/raw	Frozen	Canned	Processed/packaged	
Prepared by others	Other (Explain)			

Beverage Consumed:

Soda   Diet soda/seltzer water   Tap/bottled water
Milk/dairy alternative Other (Explain)

Exercise Location and Activity:

Level of Activity: Easy   Moderate   Vigorous   Highly Vigorous

Who joined you: **Or Circle:**   Ate Alone/Exercised Alone

Feelings experienced before/during/after and how you responded to those feelings? Were they expressed in the session? If so, how and if not, why not?

What positive step did you take or guardrail did you apply during this session? Did it go as planned? Would you do anything differently next time?

ACTIVITY REFLECTION

Journal some thoughts about the meal or snack you selected or the exercise you undertook. How did the meal/snack look, smell, and taste? What did you notice going on around you as you exercised? How were you in control of this session and how did this session control you?

EMOTION REFLECTION

Journal about the feelings you experienced and how you responded to them. Was this session a reflection of feelings and emotions? List some positive self-talk responses you can offer to your internal critic to combat the lies you hear in your head.

When you complete your last session of Day 30, move on to the Phase Three Reflection.

Phase Three Session Log Sheet

Day 21 - Day 30

Complete the log for this food/exercise session. Place a checkmark next to or circle all that apply.

Date: **Day of Week**:   **Time**:   AM/PM

Reason for the session: Meal   Snack   Exercise   Other (Explain)

Meal Components: Protein   Fruit   Whole grain   Vegetable   Healthy Fat

Method of Preparation:

Baked	Broiled	Sautéed	Grilled	Boiled
Fried	Roasted	Steamed	Stir-fry	Stewed
Fresh/raw	Frozen	Canned	Processed/packaged	
Prepared by others	Other (Explain)			

Beverage Consumed:

Soda	Diet soda/seltzer water	Tap/bottled water
Milk/dairy alternative	Other (Explain)	

Exercise Location and Activity:

Level of Activity: Easy   Moderate   Vigorous   Highly Vigorous

Who joined you: **Or Circle:**   Ate Alone/Exercised Alone

Feelings experienced before/during/after and how you responded to those feelings? Were they expressed in the session? If so, how and if not, why not?

What positive step did you take or guardrail did you apply during this session? Did it go as planned? Would you do anything differently next time?

ACTIVITY REFLECTION

Journal some thoughts about the meal or snack you selected or the exercise you undertook. How did the meal/snack look, smell, and taste? What did you notice going on around you as you exercised? How were you in control of this session and how did this session control you?

EMOTION REFLECTION

Journal about the feelings you experienced and how you responded to them. Was this session a reflection of feelings and emotions? List some positive self-talk responses you can offer to your internal critic to combat the lies you hear in your head.

When you complete your last session of Day 30, move on to the Phase Three Reflection.

Phase Three Session Log Sheet

Day 21 - Day 30

Complete the log for this food/exercise session. Place a checkmark next to or circle all that apply.

Date: **Day of Week:**   **Time:**   AM/PM

Reason for the session: Meal   Snack   Exercise   Other (Explain)

Meal Components: Protein   Fruit   Whole grain   Vegetable   Healthy Fat

Method of Preparation:

Baked	Broiled	Sautéed	Grilled	Boiled
Fried	Roasted	Steamed	Stir-fry	Stewed
Fresh/raw	Frozen	Canned	Processed/packaged	
Prepared by others	Other (Explain)			

Beverage Consumed:

Soda   Diet soda/seltzer water   Tap/bottled water
Milk/dairy alternative Other (Explain)

Exercise Location and Activity:

Level of Activity: Easy   Moderate   Vigorous   Highly Vigorous

Who joined you: **Or Circle:**   Ate Alone/Exercised Alone

Feelings experienced before/during/after and how you responded to those feelings? Were they expressed in the session? If so, how and if not, why not?

What positive step did you take or guardrail did you apply during this session? Did it go as planned? Would you do anything differently next time?

ACTIVITY REFLECTION

Journal some thoughts about the meal or snack you selected or the exercise you undertook. How did the meal/snack look, smell, and taste? What did you notice going on around you as you exercised? How were you in control of this session and how did this session control you?

EMOTION REFLECTION

Journal about the feelings you experienced and how you responded to them. Was this session a reflection of feelings and emotions? List some positive self-talk responses you can offer to your internal critic to combat the lies you hear in your head.

When you complete your last session of Day 30, move on to the Phase Three Reflection.

Phase Three Session Log Sheet

Day 21 - Day 30

Complete the log for this food/exercise session. Place a checkmark next to or circle all that apply.

Date: **Day of Week:** **Time:** AM/PM

Reason for the session: Meal Snack Exercise Other (Explain)

Meal Components: Protein Fruit Whole grain Vegetable Healthy Fat

Method of Preparation:

Baked	Broiled	Sautéed	Grilled	Boiled
Fried	Roasted	Steamed	Stir-fry	Stewed
Fresh/raw	Frozen	Canned	Processed/packaged	
Prepared by others	Other (Explain)			

Beverage Consumed:

Soda Diet soda/seltzer water Tap/bottled water
Milk/dairy alternative Other (Explain)

Exercise Location and Activity:

Level of Activity: Easy Moderate Vigorous Highly Vigorous

Who joined you: **Or Circle:** Ate Alone/Exercised Alone

Feelings experienced before/during/after and how you responded to those feelings? Were they expressed in the session? If so, how and if not, why not?

What positive step did you take or guardrail did you apply during this session? Did it go as planned? Would you do anything differently next time?

ACTIVITY REFLECTION

Journal some thoughts about the meal or snack you selected or the exercise you undertook. How did the meal/snack look, smell, and taste? What did you notice going on around you as you exercised? How were you in control of this session and how did this session control you?

EMOTION REFLECTION

Journal about the feelings you experienced and how you responded to them. Was this session a reflection of feelings and emotions? List some positive self-talk responses you can offer to your internal critic to combat the lies you hear in your head.

When you complete your last session of Day 30, move on to the Phase Three Reflection.

Phase Three Session Log Sheet

Day 21 - Day 30

Complete the log for this food/exercise session. Place a checkmark next to or circle all that apply.

Date: **Day of Week:** **Time:** AM/PM

Reason for the session: Meal   Snack   Exercise   Other (Explain)

Meal Components: Protein   Fruit   Whole grain   Vegetable   Healthy Fat

Method of Preparation:

Baked	Broiled	Sautéed	Grilled	Boiled
Fried	Roasted	Steamed	Stir-fry	Stewed
Fresh/raw	Frozen	Canned	Processed/packaged	
Prepared by others	Other (Explain)			

Beverage Consumed:

Soda   Diet soda/seltzer water   Tap/bottled water
Milk/dairy alternative   Other (Explain)

Exercise Location and Activity:

Level of Activity: Easy   Moderate   Vigorous   Highly Vigorous

Who joined you: **Or Circle:**   Ate Alone/Exercised Alone

Feelings experienced before/during/after and how you responded to those feelings? Were they expressed in the session? If so, how and if not, why not?

What positive step did you take or guardrail did you apply during this session? Did it go as planned? Would you do anything differently next time?

Activity Reflection

Journal some thoughts about the meal or snack you selected or the exercise you undertook. How did the meal/snack look, smell, and taste? What did you notice going on around you as you exercised? How were you in control of this session and how did this session control you?

Emotion Reflection

Journal about the feelings you experienced and how you responded to them. Was this session a reflection of feelings and emotions? List some positive self-talk responses you can offer to your internal critic to combat the lies you hear in your head.

When you complete your last session of Day 30, move on to the Phase Three Reflection.

Phase Three Session Log Sheet

Day 21 - Day 30

Complete the log for this food/exercise session. Place a checkmark next to or circle all that apply.

Date: **Day of Week:** **Time:** AM/PM

Reason for the session: Meal Snack Exercise Other (Explain)

Meal Components: Protein Fruit Whole grain Vegetable Healthy Fat

Method of Preparation:

Baked	Broiled	Sautéed	Grilled	Boiled
Fried	Roasted	Steamed	Stir-fry	Stewed
Fresh/raw	Frozen	Canned	Processed/packaged	
Prepared by others	Other (Explain)			

Beverage Consumed:

Soda Diet soda/seltzer water Tap/bottled water
Milk/dairy alternative Other (Explain)

Exercise Location and Activity:

Level of Activity: Easy Moderate Vigorous Highly Vigorous

Who joined you: **Or Circle:** Ate Alone/Exercised Alone

Feelings experienced before/during/after and how you responded to those feelings? Were they expressed in the session? If so, how and if not, why not?

What positive step did you take or guardrail did you apply during this session? Did it go as planned? Would you do anything differently next time?

ACTIVITY REFLECTION

Journal some thoughts about the meal or snack you selected or the exercise you undertook. How did the meal/snack look, smell, and taste? What did you notice going on around you as you exercised? How were you in control of this session and how did this session control you?

EMOTION REFLECTION

Journal about the feelings you experienced and how you responded to them. Was this session a reflection of feelings and emotions? List some positive self-talk responses you can offer to your internal critic to combat the lies you hear in your head.

When you complete your last session of Day 30, move on to the Phase Three Reflection.

Phase Three Session Log Sheet

Day 21 - Day 30

Complete the log for this food/exercise session. Place a checkmark next to or circle all that apply.

Date: **Day of Week**:   **Time**:   AM/PM

Reason for the session: Meal   Snack   Exercise   Other (Explain)

Meal Components: Protein   Fruit   Whole grain   Vegetable   Healthy Fat

Method of Preparation:

Baked	Broiled	Sautéed	Grilled	Boiled
Fried	Roasted	Steamed	Stir-fry	Stewed
Fresh/raw	Frozen	Canned	Processed/packaged	
Prepared by others	Other (Explain)			

Beverage Consumed:

Soda	Diet soda/seltzer water	Tap/bottled water
Milk/dairy alternative	Other (Explain)	

Exercise Location and Activity:

Level of Activity: Easy   Moderate   Vigorous   Highly Vigorous

Who joined you: **Or Circle**:   Ate Alone/Exercised Alone

Feelings experienced before/during/after and how you responded to those feelings? Were they expressed in the session? If so, how and if not, why not?

What positive step did you take or guardrail did you apply during this session? Did it go as planned? Would you do anything differently next time?

Activity Reflection

Journal some thoughts about the meal or snack you selected or the exercise you undertook. How did the meal/snack look, smell, and taste? What did you notice going on around you as you exercised? How were you in control of this session and how did this session control you?

Emotion Reflection

Journal about the feelings you experienced and how you responded to them. Was this session a reflection of feelings and emotions? List some positive self-talk responses you can offer to your internal critic to combat the lies you hear in your head.

When you complete your last session of Day 30, move on to the Phase Three Reflection.

Phase Three Session Log Sheet

Day 21 - Day 30

Complete the log for this food/exercise session. Place a checkmark next to or circle all that apply.

Date:　　　　　　　　**Day of Week**:　　　　　　　　**Time**:　　　　　AM/PM

Reason for the session:　　Meal　　　　Snack　　　　Exercise　　　　Other (Explain)

Meal Components:　　Protein　　Fruit　　Whole grain　　Vegetable　　Healthy Fat

Method of Preparation:

Baked	Broiled	Sautéed	Grilled	Boiled
Fried	Roasted	Steamed	Stir-fry	Stewed
Fresh/raw	Frozen	Canned	Processed/packaged	
Prepared by others	Other (Explain)			

Beverage Consumed:

Soda	Diet soda/seltzer water	Tap/bottled water
Milk/dairy alternative	Other (Explain)	

Exercise Location and Activity:

Level of Activity:　　　　Easy　　　　Moderate　　　　Vigorous　　　　Highly Vigorous

Who joined you:　　　　　　　　**Or Circle**:　　　　Ate Alone/Exercised Alone

Feelings experienced before/during/after and how you responded to those feelings? Were they expressed in the session? If so, how and if not, why not?

What positive step did you take or guardrail did you apply during this session? Did it go as planned? Would you do anything differently next time?

Activity Reflection

Journal some thoughts about the meal or snack you selected or the exercise you undertook. How did the meal/snack look, smell, and taste? What did you notice going on around you as you exercised? How were you in control of this session and how did this session control you?

Emotion Reflection

Journal about the feelings you experienced and how you responded to them. Was this session a reflection of feelings and emotions? List some positive self-talk responses you can offer to your internal critic to combat the lies you hear in your head.

When you complete your last session of Day 30, move on to the Phase Three Reflection.

Phase Three Session Log Sheet

Day 21 - Day 30

Complete the log for this food/exercise session. Place a checkmark next to or circle all that apply.

Date: **Day of Week:**   **Time:**   AM/PM

Reason for the session: Meal   Snack   Exercise   Other (Explain)

Meal Components: Protein   Fruit   Whole grain   Vegetable   Healthy Fat

Method of Preparation:

Baked	Broiled	Sautéed	Grilled	Boiled
Fried	Roasted	Steamed	Stir-fry	Stewed
Fresh/raw	Frozen	Canned	Processed/packaged	
Prepared by others	Other (Explain)			

Beverage Consumed:

Soda   Diet soda/seltzer water   Tap/bottled water
Milk/dairy alternative Other (Explain)

Exercise Location and Activity:

Level of Activity: Easy   Moderate   Vigorous   Highly Vigorous

Who joined you: **Or Circle:**   Ate Alone/Exercised Alone

Feelings experienced before/during/after and how you responded to those feelings? Were they expressed in the session? If so, how and if not, why not?

What positive step did you take or guardrail did you apply during this session? Did it go as planned? Would you do anything differently next time?

ACTIVITY REFLECTION

Journal some thoughts about the meal or snack you selected or the exercise you undertook. How did the meal/snack look, smell, and taste? What did you notice going on around you as you exercised? How were you in control of this session and how did this session control you?

EMOTION REFLECTION

Journal about the feelings you experienced and how you responded to them. Was this session a reflection of feelings and emotions? List some positive self-talk responses you can offer to your internal critic to combat the lies you hear in your head.

When you complete your last session of Day 30, move on to the Phase Three Reflection.

Phase Three Session Log Sheet

Day 21 - Day 30

Complete the log for this food/exercise session. Place a checkmark next to or circle all that apply.

Date: **Day of Week:** **Time:** AM/PM

Reason for the session: Meal Snack Exercise Other (Explain)

Meal Components: Protein Fruit Whole grain Vegetable Healthy Fat

Method of Preparation:

Baked	Broiled	Sautéed	Grilled	Boiled
Fried	Roasted	Steamed	Stir-fry	Stewed
Fresh/raw	Frozen	Canned	Processed/packaged	
Prepared by others	Other (Explain)			

Beverage Consumed:

Soda   Diet soda/seltzer water   Tap/bottled water
Milk/dairy alternative   Other (Explain)

Exercise Location and Activity:

Level of Activity: Easy Moderate Vigorous Highly Vigorous

Who joined you: **Or Circle:** Ate Alone/Exercised Alone

Feelings experienced before/during/after and how you responded to those feelings? Were they expressed in the session? If so, how and if not, why not?

What positive step did you take or guardrail did you apply during this session? Did it go as planned? Would you do anything differently next time?

ACTIVITY REFLECTION

Journal some thoughts about the meal or snack you selected or the exercise you undertook. How did the meal/snack look, smell, and taste? What did you notice going on around you as you exercised? How were you in control of this session and how did this session control you?

EMOTION REFLECTION

Journal about the feelings you experienced and how you responded to them. Was this session a reflection of feelings and emotions? List some positive self-talk responses you can offer to your internal critic to combat the lies you hear in your head.

When you complete your last session of Day 30, move on to the Phase Three Reflection.

Phase Three Session Log Sheet

Day 21 - Day 30

Complete the log for this food/exercise session. Place a checkmark next to or circle all that apply.

Date: **Day of Week:** **Time:** AM/PM

Reason for the session: Meal   Snack   Exercise   Other (Explain)

Meal Components: Protein   Fruit   Whole grain   Vegetable   Healthy Fat

Method of Preparation:

Baked	Broiled	Sautéed	Grilled	Boiled
Fried	Roasted	Steamed	Stir-fry	Stewed
Fresh/raw	Frozen	Canned	Processed/packaged	
Prepared by others	Other (Explain)			

Beverage Consumed:

Soda   Diet soda/seltzer water   Tap/bottled water
Milk/dairy alternative   Other (Explain)

Exercise Location and Activity:

Level of Activity: Easy   Moderate   Vigorous   Highly Vigorous

Who joined you: **Or Circle:**   Ate Alone/Exercised Alone

Feelings experienced before/during/after and how you responded to those feelings? Were they expressed in the session? If so, how and if not, why not?

What positive step did you take or guardrail did you apply during this session? Did it go as planned? Would you do anything differently next time?

Activity Reflection

Journal some thoughts about the meal or snack you selected or the exercise you undertook. How did the meal/snack look, smell, and taste? What did you notice going on around you as you exercised? How were you in control of this session and how did this session control you?

Emotion Reflection

Journal about the feelings you experienced and how you responded to them. Was this session a reflection of feelings and emotions? List some positive self-talk responses you can offer to your internal critic to combat the lies you hear in your head.

When you complete your last session of Day 30, move on to the Phase Three Reflection.

Phase Three Session Log Sheet

Day 21 - Day 30

Complete the log for this food/exercise session. Place a checkmark next to or circle all that apply.

Date:	**Day of Week**:	**Time**:	AM/PM

Reason for the session:	Meal	Snack	Exercise	Other (Explain)

Meal Components:	Protein	Fruit	Whole grain	Vegetable	Healthy Fat

Method of Preparation:

Baked	Broiled	Sautéed	Grilled	Boiled
Fried	Roasted	Steamed	Stir-fry	Stewed
Fresh/raw	Frozen	Canned	Processed/packaged	
Prepared by others	Other (Explain)			

Beverage Consumed:

Soda	Diet soda/seltzer water	Tap/bottled water
Milk/dairy alternative	Other (Explain)	

Exercise Location and Activity:

Level of Activity:	Easy	Moderate	Vigorous	Highly Vigorous

Who joined you:		**Or Circle**:	Ate Alone/Exercised Alone

Feelings experienced before/during/after and how you responded to those feelings? Were they expressed in the session? If so, how and if not, why not?

What positive step did you take or guardrail did you apply during this session? Did it go as planned? Would you do anything differently next time?

ACTIVITY REFLECTION

Journal some thoughts about the meal or snack you selected or the exercise you undertook. How did the meal/snack look, smell, and taste? What did you notice going on around you as you exercised? How were you in control of this session and how did this session control you?

EMOTION REFLECTION

Journal about the feelings you experienced and how you responded to them. Was this session a reflection of feelings and emotions? List some positive self-talk responses you can offer to your internal critic to combat the lies you hear in your head.

When you complete your last session of Day 30, move on to the Phase Three Reflection.

Phase Three Session Log Sheet

Day 21 - Day 30

Complete the log for this food/exercise session. Place a checkmark next to or circle all that apply.

Date: **Day of Week:** **Time:** AM/PM

Reason for the session: Meal Snack Exercise Other (Explain)

Meal Components: Protein Fruit Whole grain Vegetable Healthy Fat

Method of Preparation:

Baked	Broiled	Sautéed	Grilled	Boiled
Fried	Roasted	Steamed	Stir-fry	Stewed
Fresh/raw	Frozen	Canned	Processed/packaged	
Prepared by others	Other (Explain)			

Beverage Consumed:

Soda Diet soda/seltzer water Tap/bottled water
Milk/dairy alternative Other (Explain)

Exercise Location and Activity:

Level of Activity: Easy Moderate Vigorous Highly Vigorous

Who joined you: **Or Circle:** Ate Alone/Exercised Alone

Feelings experienced before/during/after and how you responded to those feelings? Were they expressed in the session? If so, how and if not, why not?

What positive step did you take or guardrail did you apply during this session? Did it go as planned? Would you do anything differently next time?

Activity Reflection

Journal some thoughts about the meal or snack you selected or the exercise you undertook. How did the meal/snack look, smell, and taste? What did you notice going on around you as you exercised? How were you in control of this session and how did this session control you?

Emotion Reflection

Journal about the feelings you experienced and how you responded to them. Was this session a reflection of feelings and emotions? List some positive self-talk responses you can offer to your internal critic to combat the lies you hear in your head.

When you complete your last session of Day 30, move on to the Phase Three Reflection.

Phase Three Session Log Sheet

Day 21 - Day 30

Complete the log for this food/exercise session. Place a checkmark next to or circle all that apply.

Date: **Day of Week:** **Time:** AM/PM

Reason for the session: Meal Snack Exercise Other (Explain)

Meal Components: Protein Fruit Whole grain Vegetable Healthy Fat

Method of Preparation:

Baked	Broiled	Sautéed	Grilled	Boiled
Fried	Roasted	Steamed	Stir-fry	Stewed
Fresh/raw	Frozen	Canned	Processed/packaged	
Prepared by others	Other (Explain)			

Beverage Consumed:

Soda Diet soda/seltzer water Tap/bottled water
Milk/dairy alternative Other (Explain)

Exercise Location and Activity:

Level of Activity: Easy Moderate Vigorous Highly Vigorous

Who joined you: **Or Circle:** Ate Alone/Exercised Alone

Feelings experienced before/during/after and how you responded to those feelings? Were they expressed in the session? If so, how and if not, why not?

What positive step did you take or guardrail did you apply during this session? Did it go as planned? Would you do anything differently next time?

ACTIVITY REFLECTION

Journal some thoughts about the meal or snack you selected or the exercise you undertook. How did the meal/snack look, smell, and taste? What did you notice going on around you as you exercised? How were you in control of this session and how did this session control you?

EMOTION REFLECTION

Journal about the feelings you experienced and how you responded to them. Was this session a reflection of feelings and emotions? List some positive self-talk responses you can offer to your internal critic to combat the lies you hear in your head.

When you complete your last session of Day 30, move on to the Phase Three Reflection.

Phase Three Session Log Sheet

Day 21 - Day 30

Complete the log for this food/exercise session. Place a checkmark next to or circle all that apply.

Date: **Day of Week**:   **Time**:   AM/PM

Reason for the session: Meal   Snack   Exercise   Other (Explain)

Meal Components: Protein   Fruit   Whole grain   Vegetable   Healthy Fat

Method of Preparation:

Baked	Broiled	Sautéed	Grilled	Boiled
Fried	Roasted	Steamed	Stir-fry	Stewed
Fresh/raw	Frozen	Canned	Processed/packaged	
Prepared by others	Other (Explain)			

Beverage Consumed:

Soda	Diet soda/seltzer water	Tap/bottled water
Milk/dairy alternative	Other (Explain)	

Exercise Location and Activity:

Level of Activity: Easy   Moderate   Vigorous   Highly Vigorous

Who joined you: **Or Circle:**   Ate Alone/Exercised Alone

Feelings experienced before/during/after and how you responded to those feelings? Were they expressed in the session? If so, how and if not, why not?

What positive step did you take or guardrail did you apply during this session? Did it go as planned? Would you do anything differently next time?

ACTIVITY REFLECTION

Journal some thoughts about the meal or snack you selected or the exercise you undertook. How did the meal/snack look, smell, and taste? What did you notice going on around you as you exercised? How were you in control of this session and how did this session control you?

EMOTION REFLECTION

Journal about the feelings you experienced and how you responded to them. Was this session a reflection of feelings and emotions? List some positive self-talk responses you can offer to your internal critic to combat the lies you hear in your head.

When you complete your last session of Day 30, move on to the Phase Three Reflection.

Phase Three Session Log Sheet

Day 21 - Day 30

Complete the log for this food/exercise session. Place a checkmark next to or circle all that apply.

Date:　　　　　　　　**Day of Week:**　　　　　　　**Time:**　　　　　AM/PM

Reason for the session:　　Meal　　　　Snack　　　　Exercise　　　　Other (Explain)

Meal Components:　　Protein　　Fruit　　Whole grain　　Vegetable　　Healthy Fat

Method of Preparation:

Baked	Broiled	Sautéed	Grilled	Boiled
Fried	Roasted	Steamed	Stir-fry	Stewed
Fresh/raw	Frozen	Canned	Processed/packaged	
Prepared by others	Other (Explain)			

Beverage Consumed:

Soda	Diet soda/seltzer water	Tap/bottled water
Milk/dairy alternative	Other (Explain)	

Exercise Location and Activity:

Level of Activity:　　　　Easy　　　　Moderate　　　　Vigorous　　　　Highly Vigorous

Who joined you:　　　　　　　　**Or Circle:**　　　　Ate Alone/Exercised Alone

Feelings experienced before/during/after and how you responded to those feelings? Were they expressed in the session? If so, how and if not, why not?

What positive step did you take or guardrail did you apply during this session? Did it go as planned? Would you do anything differently next time?

ACTIVITY REFLECTION

Journal some thoughts about the meal or snack you selected or the exercise you undertook. How did the meal/snack look, smell, and taste? What did you notice going on around you as you exercised? How were you in control of this session and how did this session control you?

EMOTION REFLECTION

Journal about the feelings you experienced and how you responded to them. Was this session a reflection of feelings and emotions? List some positive self-talk responses you can offer to your internal critic to combat the lies you hear in your head.

When you complete your last session of Day 30, move on to the Phase Three Reflection.

Phase Three Session Log Sheet

Day 21 - Day 30

Complete the log for this food/exercise session. Place a checkmark next to or circle all that apply.

Date: **Day of Week**:   **Time**:   AM/PM

Reason for the session: Meal   Snack   Exercise   Other (Explain)

Meal Components: Protein   Fruit   Whole grain   Vegetable   Healthy Fat

Method of Preparation:

Baked	Broiled	Sautéed	Grilled	Boiled
Fried	Roasted	Steamed	Stir-fry	Stewed
Fresh/raw	Frozen	Canned	Processed/packaged	
Prepared by others	Other (Explain)			

Beverage Consumed:

Soda   Diet soda/seltzer water   Tap/bottled water
Milk/dairy alternative   Other (Explain)

Exercise Location and Activity:

Level of Activity: Easy   Moderate   Vigorous   Highly Vigorous

Who joined you: **Or Circle**:   Ate Alone/Exercised Alone

Feelings experienced before/during/after and how you responded to those feelings? Were they expressed in the session? If so, how and if not, why not?

What positive step did you take or guardrail did you apply during this session? Did it go as planned? Would you do anything differently next time?

Activity Reflection

Journal some thoughts about the meal or snack you selected or the exercise you undertook. How did the meal/snack look, smell, and taste? What did you notice going on around you as you exercised? How were you in control of this session and how did this session control you?

Emotion Reflection

Journal about the feelings you experienced and how you responded to them. Was this session a reflection of feelings and emotions? List some positive self-talk responses you can offer to your internal critic to combat the lies you hear in your head.

When you complete your last session of Day 30, move on to the Phase Three Reflection.

Phase Three Session Log Sheet

Day 21 - Day 30

Complete the log for this food/exercise session. Place a checkmark next to or circle all that apply.

Date: **Day of Week**:   **Time**:   AM/PM

Reason for the session: Meal   Snack   Exercise   Other (Explain)

Meal Components: Protein   Fruit   Whole grain   Vegetable   Healthy Fat

Method of Preparation:

Baked	Broiled	Sautéed	Grilled	Boiled
Fried	Roasted	Steamed	Stir-fry	Stewed
Fresh/raw	Frozen	Canned	Processed/packaged	
Prepared by others	Other (Explain)			

Beverage Consumed:

Soda   Diet soda/seltzer water   Tap/bottled water
Milk/dairy alternative   Other (Explain)

Exercise Location and Activity:

Level of Activity: Easy   Moderate   Vigorous   Highly Vigorous

Who joined you: **Or Circle**:   Ate Alone/Exercised Alone

Feelings experienced before/during/after and how you responded to those feelings? Were they expressed in the session? If so, how and if not, why not?

What positive step did you take or guardrail did you apply during this session? Did it go as planned? Would you do anything differently next time?

ACTIVITY REFLECTION

Journal some thoughts about the meal or snack you selected or the exercise you undertook. How did the meal/snack look, smell, and taste? What did you notice going on around you as you exercised? How were you in control of this session and how did this session control you?

EMOTION REFLECTION

Journal about the feelings you experienced and how you responded to them. Was this session a reflection of feelings and emotions? List some positive self-talk responses you can offer to your internal critic to combat the lies you hear in your head.

When you complete your last session of Day 30, move on to the Phase Three Reflection.

Phase Three Session Log Sheet

Day 21 - Day 30

Complete the log for this food/exercise session. Place a checkmark next to or circle all that apply.

Date: **Day of Week:** **Time:** AM/PM

Reason for the session: Meal Snack Exercise Other (Explain)

Meal Components: Protein Fruit Whole grain Vegetable Healthy Fat

Method of Preparation:

Baked	Broiled	Sautéed	Grilled	Boiled
Fried	Roasted	Steamed	Stir-fry	Stewed
Fresh/raw	Frozen	Canned	Processed/packaged	
Prepared by others	Other (Explain)			

Beverage Consumed:

Soda Diet soda/seltzer water Tap/bottled water
Milk/dairy alternative Other (Explain)

Exercise Location and Activity:

Level of Activity: Easy Moderate Vigorous Highly Vigorous

Who joined you: **Or Circle:** Ate Alone/Exercised Alone

Feelings experienced before/during/after and how you responded to those feelings? Were they expressed in the session? If so, how and if not, why not?

What positive step did you take or guardrail did you apply during this session? Did it go as planned? Would you do anything differently next time?

ACTIVITY REFLECTION

Journal some thoughts about the meal or snack you selected or the exercise you undertook. How did the meal/snack look, smell, and taste? What did you notice going on around you as you exercised? How were you in control of this session and how did this session control you?

EMOTION REFLECTION

Journal about the feelings you experienced and how you responded to them. Was this session a reflection of feelings and emotions? List some positive self-talk responses you can offer to your internal critic to combat the lies you hear in your head.

When you complete your last session of Day 30, move on to the Phase Three Reflection.

Phase Three Session Log Sheet

Day 21 - Day 30

Complete the log for this food/exercise session. Place a checkmark next to or circle all that apply.

Date:　　　　　　　　**Day of Week**:　　　　　　　　**Time**:　　　　　AM/PM

Reason for the session:　　Meal　　　　Snack　　　　Exercise　　　　Other (Explain)

Meal Components:　　Protein　　Fruit　　Whole grain　　Vegetable　　Healthy Fat

Method of Preparation:

Baked	Broiled	Sautéed	Grilled	Boiled
Fried	Roasted	Steamed	Stir-fry	Stewed
Fresh/raw	Frozen	Canned	Processed/packaged	
Prepared by others	Other (Explain)			

Beverage Consumed:

Soda	Diet soda/seltzer water	Tap/bottled water
Milk/dairy alternative	Other (Explain)	

Exercise Location and Activity:

Level of Activity:　　　　Easy　　　　Moderate　　　　Vigorous　　　　Highly Vigorous

Who joined you:　　　　　　　　**Or Circle**:　　　　Ate Alone/Exercised Alone

Feelings experienced before/during/after and how you responded to those feelings? Were they expressed in the session? If so, how and if not, why not?

What positive step did you take or guardrail did you apply during this session? Did it go as planned? Would you do anything differently next time?

ACTIVITY REFLECTION

Journal some thoughts about the meal or snack you selected or the exercise you undertook. How did the meal/snack look, smell, and taste? What did you notice going on around you as you exercised? How were you in control of this session and how did this session control you?

EMOTION REFLECTION

Journal about the feelings you experienced and how you responded to them. Was this session a reflection of feelings and emotions? List some positive self-talk responses you can offer to your internal critic to combat the lies you hear in your head.

When you complete your last session of Day 30, move on to the Phase Three Reflection.

Phase Three Session Log Sheet

Day 21 - Day 30

Complete the log for this food/exercise session. Place a checkmark next to or circle all that apply.

Date: **Day of Week:**   **Time:**   AM/PM

Reason for the session: Meal   Snack   Exercise   Other (Explain)

Meal Components: Protein   Fruit   Whole grain   Vegetable   Healthy Fat

Method of Preparation:

Baked	Broiled	Sautéed	Grilled	Boiled
Fried	Roasted	Steamed	Stir-fry	Stewed
Fresh/raw	Frozen	Canned	Processed/packaged	
Prepared by others	Other (Explain)			

Beverage Consumed:

Soda   Diet soda/seltzer water   Tap/bottled water
Milk/dairy alternative   Other (Explain)

Exercise Location and Activity:

Level of Activity: Easy   Moderate   Vigorous   Highly Vigorous

Who joined you: **Or Circle:**   Ate Alone/Exercised Alone

Feelings experienced before/during/after and how you responded to those feelings? Were they expressed in the session? If so, how and if not, why not?

What positive step did you take or guardrail did you apply during this session? Did it go as planned? Would you do anything differently next time?

ACTIVITY REFLECTION

Journal some thoughts about the meal or snack you selected or the exercise you undertook. How did the meal/snack look, smell, and taste? What did you notice going on around you as you exercised? How were you in control of this session and how did this session control you?

EMOTION REFLECTION

Journal about the feelings you experienced and how you responded to them. Was this session a reflection of feelings and emotions? List some positive self-talk responses you can offer to your internal critic to combat the lies you hear in your head.

When you complete your last session of Day 30, move on to the Phase Three Reflection.

Phase Three Session Log Sheet

Day 21 - Day 30

Complete the log for this food/exercise session. Place a checkmark next to or circle all that apply.

Date: **Day of Week**:   **Time**:   AM/PM

Reason for the session: Meal   Snack   Exercise   Other (Explain)

Meal Components: Protein   Fruit   Whole grain   Vegetable   Healthy Fat

Method of Preparation:

Baked	Broiled	Sautéed	Grilled	Boiled
Fried	Roasted	Steamed	Stir-fry	Stewed
Fresh/raw	Frozen	Canned	Processed/packaged	
Prepared by others	Other (Explain)			

Beverage Consumed:

Soda   Diet soda/seltzer water   Tap/bottled water
Milk/dairy alternative Other (Explain)

Exercise Location and Activity:

Level of Activity: Easy   Moderate   Vigorous   Highly Vigorous

Who joined you: **Or Circle**:   Ate Alone/Exercised Alone

Feelings experienced before/during/after and how you responded to those feelings? Were they expressed in the session? If so, how and if not, why not?

What positive step did you take or guardrail did you apply during this session? Did it go as planned? Would you do anything differently next time?

Activity Reflection

Journal some thoughts about the meal or snack you selected or the exercise you undertook. How did the meal/snack look, smell, and taste? What did you notice going on around you as you exercised? How were you in control of this session and how did this session control you?

Emotion Reflection

Journal about the feelings you experienced and how you responded to them. Was this session a reflection of feelings and emotions? List some positive self-talk responses you can offer to your internal critic to combat the lies you hear in your head.

When you complete your last session of Day 30, move on to the Phase Three Reflection.

Phase Three Session Log Sheet

Day 21 - Day 30

Complete the log for this food/exercise session. Place a checkmark next to or circle all that apply.

Date: **Day of Week**:   **Time**:   AM/PM

Reason for the session: Meal   Snack   Exercise   Other (Explain)

Meal Components: Protein   Fruit   Whole grain   Vegetable   Healthy Fat

Method of Preparation:

Baked	Broiled	Sautéed	Grilled	Boiled
Fried	Roasted	Steamed	Stir-fry	Stewed
Fresh/raw	Frozen	Canned	Processed/packaged	
Prepared by others	Other (Explain)			

Beverage Consumed:

Soda   Diet soda/seltzer water   Tap/bottled water
Milk/dairy alternative Other (Explain)

Exercise Location and Activity:

Level of Activity: Easy   Moderate   Vigorous   Highly Vigorous

Who joined you: **Or Circle:**   Ate Alone/Exercised Alone

Feelings experienced before/during/after and how you responded to those feelings? Were they expressed in the session? If so, how and if not, why not?

What positive step did you take or guardrail did you apply during this session? Did it go as planned? Would you do anything differently next time?

ACTIVITY REFLECTION

Journal some thoughts about the meal or snack you selected or the exercise you undertook. How did the meal/snack look, smell, and taste? What did you notice going on around you as you exercised? How were you in control of this session and how did this session control you?

EMOTION REFLECTION

Journal about the feelings you experienced and how you responded to them. Was this session a reflection of feelings and emotions? List some positive self-talk responses you can offer to your internal critic to combat the lies you hear in your head.

When you complete your last session of Day 30, move on to the Phase Three Reflection.

Phase Three Session Log Sheet

Day 21 - Day 30

Complete the log for this food/exercise session. Place a checkmark next to or circle all that apply.

Date: **Day of Week:**   **Time:**   AM/PM

Reason for the session: Meal   Snack   Exercise   Other (Explain)

Meal Components: Protein   Fruit   Whole grain   Vegetable   Healthy Fat

Method of Preparation:

Baked	Broiled	Sautéed	Grilled	Boiled
Fried	Roasted	Steamed	Stir-fry	Stewed
Fresh/raw	Frozen	Canned	Processed/packaged	
Prepared by others	Other (Explain)			

Beverage Consumed:

Soda	Diet soda/seltzer water	Tap/bottled water
Milk/dairy alternative	Other (Explain)	

Exercise Location and Activity:

Level of Activity: Easy   Moderate   Vigorous   Highly Vigorous

Who joined you: **Or Circle:**   Ate Alone/Exercised Alone

Feelings experienced before/during/after and how you responded to those feelings? Were they expressed in the session? If so, how and if not, why not?

What positive step did you take or guardrail did you apply during this session? Did it go as planned? Would you do anything differently next time?

ACTIVITY REFLECTION

Journal some thoughts about the meal or snack you selected or the exercise you undertook. How did the meal/snack look, smell, and taste? What did you notice going on around you as you exercised? How were you in control of this session and how did this session control you?

EMOTION REFLECTION

Journal about the feelings you experienced and how you responded to them. Was this session a reflection of feelings and emotions? List some positive self-talk responses you can offer to your internal critic to combat the lies you hear in your head.

When you complete your last session of Day 30, move on to the Phase Three Reflection.

Phase Three Session Log Sheet

Day 21 - Day 30

Complete the log for this food/exercise session. Place a checkmark next to or circle all that apply.

Date: **Day of Week**:   **Time**:   AM/PM

Reason for the session: Meal   Snack   Exercise   Other (Explain)

Meal Components: Protein   Fruit   Whole grain   Vegetable   Healthy Fat

Method of Preparation:

Baked	Broiled	Sautéed	Grilled	Boiled
Fried	Roasted	Steamed	Stir-fry	Stewed
Fresh/raw	Frozen	Canned	Processed/packaged	
Prepared by others	Other (Explain)			

Beverage Consumed:

Soda   Diet soda/seltzer water   Tap/bottled water
Milk/dairy alternative   Other (Explain)

Exercise Location and Activity:

Level of Activity: Easy   Moderate   Vigorous   Highly Vigorous

Who joined you: **Or Circle:**   Ate Alone/Exercised Alone

Feelings experienced before/during/after and how you responded to those feelings? Were they expressed in the session? If so, how and if not, why not?

What positive step did you take or guardrail did you apply during this session? Did it go as planned? Would you do anything differently next time?

ACTIVITY REFLECTION

Journal some thoughts about the meal or snack you selected or the exercise you undertook. How did the meal/snack look, smell, and taste? What did you notice going on around you as you exercised? How were you in control of this session and how did this session control you?

EMOTION REFLECTION

Journal about the feelings you experienced and how you responded to them. Was this session a reflection of feelings and emotions? List some positive self-talk responses you can offer to your internal critic to combat the lies you hear in your head.

When you complete your last session of Day 30, move on to the Phase Three Reflection.

Phase Three Session Log Sheet

Day 21 - Day 30

Complete the log for this food/exercise session. Place a checkmark next to or circle all that apply.

Date: **Day of Week**:   **Time**:   AM/PM

Reason for the session: Meal   Snack   Exercise   Other (Explain)

Meal Components: Protein   Fruit   Whole grain   Vegetable   Healthy Fat

Method of Preparation:

Baked	Broiled	Sautéed	Grilled	Boiled
Fried	Roasted	Steamed	Stir-fry	Stewed
Fresh/raw	Frozen	Canned	Processed/packaged	
Prepared by others	Other (Explain)			

Beverage Consumed:

Soda   Diet soda/seltzer water   Tap/bottled water
Milk/dairy alternative   Other (Explain)

Exercise Location and Activity:

Level of Activity: Easy   Moderate   Vigorous   Highly Vigorous

Who joined you: **Or Circle:**   Ate Alone/Exercised Alone

Feelings experienced before/during/after and how you responded to those feelings? Were they expressed in the session? If so, how and if not, why not?

What positive step did you take or guardrail did you apply during this session? Did it go as planned? Would you do anything differently next time?

ACTIVITY REFLECTION

Journal some thoughts about the meal or snack you selected or the exercise you undertook. How did the meal/snack look, smell, and taste? What did you notice going on around you as you exercised? How were you in control of this session and how did this session control you?

EMOTION REFLECTION

Journal about the feelings you experienced and how you responded to them. Was this session a reflection of feelings and emotions? List some positive self-talk responses you can offer to your internal critic to combat the lies you hear in your head.

When you complete your last session of Day 30, move on to the Phase Three Reflection.

Phase Three Session Log Sheet

Day 21 - Day 30

Complete the log for this food/exercise session. Place a checkmark next to or circle all that apply.

Date: **Day of Week:** **Time:** AM/PM

Reason for the session: Meal Snack Exercise Other (Explain)

Meal Components: Protein Fruit Whole grain Vegetable Healthy Fat

Method of Preparation:

Baked	Broiled	Sautéed	Grilled	Boiled
Fried	Roasted	Steamed	Stir-fry	Stewed
Fresh/raw	Frozen	Canned	Processed/packaged	
Prepared by others	Other (Explain)			

Beverage Consumed:

Soda Diet soda/seltzer water Tap/bottled water
Milk/dairy alternative Other (Explain)

Exercise Location and Activity:

Level of Activity: Easy Moderate Vigorous Highly Vigorous

Who joined you: **Or Circle:** Ate Alone/Exercised Alone

Feelings experienced before/during/after and how you responded to those feelings? Were they expressed in the session? If so, how and if not, why not?

What positive step did you take or guardrail did you apply during this session? Did it go as planned? Would you do anything differently next time?

ACTIVITY REFLECTION

Journal some thoughts about the meal or snack you selected or the exercise you undertook. How did the meal/snack look, smell, and taste? What did you notice going on around you as you exercised? How were you in control of this session and how did this session control you?

EMOTION REFLECTION

Journal about the feelings you experienced and how you responded to them. Was this session a reflection of feelings and emotions? List some positive self-talk responses you can offer to your internal critic to combat the lies you hear in your head.

When you complete your last session of Day 30, move on to the Phase Three Reflection.

Phase Three Session Log Sheet

Day 21 - Day 30

Complete the log for this food/exercise session. Place a checkmark next to or circle all that apply.

Date: **Day of Week:**   **Time:**   AM/PM

Reason for the session: Meal   Snack   Exercise   Other (Explain)

Meal Components: Protein   Fruit   Whole grain   Vegetable   Healthy Fat

Method of Preparation:

Baked	Broiled	Sautéed	Grilled	Boiled
Fried	Roasted	Steamed	Stir-fry	Stewed
Fresh/raw	Frozen	Canned	Processed/packaged	
Prepared by others	Other (Explain)			

Beverage Consumed:

Soda   Diet soda/seltzer water   Tap/bottled water
Milk/dairy alternative Other (Explain)

Exercise Location and Activity:

Level of Activity: Easy   Moderate   Vigorous   Highly Vigorous

Who joined you: **Or Circle:**   Ate Alone/Exercised Alone

Feelings experienced before/during/after and how you responded to those feelings? Were they expressed in the session? If so, how and if not, why not?

What positive step did you take or guardrail did you apply during this session? Did it go as planned? Would you do anything differently next time?

ACTIVITY REFLECTION

Journal some thoughts about the meal or snack you selected or the exercise you undertook. How did the meal/snack look, smell, and taste? What did you notice going on around you as you exercised? How were you in control of this session and how did this session control you?

EMOTION REFLECTION

Journal about the feelings you experienced and how you responded to them. Was this session a reflection of feelings and emotions? List some positive self-talk responses you can offer to your internal critic to combat the lies you hear in your head.

When you complete your last session of Day 30, move on to the Phase Three Reflection.

Phase Three Session Log Sheet

Day 21 - Day 30

Complete the log for this food/exercise session. Place a checkmark next to or circle all that apply.

Date: **Day of Week:** **Time:** AM/PM

Reason for the session:　Meal　　Snack　　Exercise　　Other (Explain)

Meal Components:　Protein　　Fruit　　Whole grain　　Vegetable　　Healthy Fat

Method of Preparation:

Baked	Broiled	Sautéed	Grilled	Boiled
Fried	Roasted	Steamed	Stir-fry	Stewed
Fresh/raw	Frozen	Canned	Processed/packaged	
Prepared by others	Other (Explain)			

Beverage Consumed:

Soda　　　　　　　　　Diet soda/seltzer water　　　　Tap/bottled water
Milk/dairy alternative　Other (Explain)

Exercise Location and Activity:

Level of Activity:　　Easy　　Moderate　　Vigorous　　Highly Vigorous

Who joined you:　　　　　　　　**Or Circle:**　　Ate Alone/Exercised Alone

Feelings experienced before/during/after and how you responded to those feelings? Were they expressed in the session? If so, how and if not, why not?

What positive step did you take or guardrail did you apply during this session? Did it go as planned? Would you do anything differently next time?

ACTIVITY REFLECTION

Journal some thoughts about the meal or snack you selected or the exercise you undertook. How did the meal/snack look, smell, and taste? What did you notice going on around you as you exercised? How were you in control of this session and how did this session control you?

EMOTION REFLECTION

Journal about the feelings you experienced and how you responded to them. Was this session a reflection of feelings and emotions? List some positive self-talk responses you can offer to your internal critic to combat the lies you hear in your head.

When you complete your last session of Day 30, move on to the Phase Three Reflection.

Phase Three Session Log Sheet

Day 21 - Day 30

Complete the log for this food/exercise session. Place a checkmark next to or circle all that apply.

Date:　　　　　　　　**Day of Week**:　　　　　　　　**Time**:　　　　AM/PM

Reason for the session:　　Meal　　　　Snack　　　　Exercise　　　　Other (Explain)

Meal Components:　　Protein　　Fruit　　Whole grain　　Vegetable　　Healthy Fat

Method of Preparation:

Baked	Broiled	Sautéed	Grilled	Boiled
Fried	Roasted	Steamed	Stir-fry	Stewed
Fresh/raw	Frozen	Canned	Processed/packaged	
Prepared by others	Other (Explain)			

Beverage Consumed:

Soda　　　　　　　　Diet soda/seltzer water　　　　Tap/bottled water
Milk/dairy alternative　　Other (Explain)

Exercise Location and Activity:

Level of Activity:　　　Easy　　　　Moderate　　　　Vigorous　　　　Highly Vigorous

Who joined you:　　　　　　　　**Or Circle**:　　　　Ate Alone/Exercised Alone

Feelings experienced before/during/after and how you responded to those feelings? Were they expressed in the session? If so, how and if not, why not?

What positive step did you take or guardrail did you apply during this session? Did it go as planned? Would you do anything differently next time?

ACTIVITY REFLECTION

Journal some thoughts about the meal or snack you selected or the exercise you undertook. How did the meal/snack look, smell, and taste? What did you notice going on around you as you exercised? How were you in control of this session and how did this session control you?

EMOTION REFLECTION

Journal about the feelings you experienced and how you responded to them. Was this session a reflection of feelings and emotions? List some positive self-talk responses you can offer to your internal critic to combat the lies you hear in your head.

When you complete your last session of Day 30, move on to the Phase Three Reflection.

Phase Three Session Log Sheet

Day 21 - Day 30

Complete the log for this food/exercise session. Place a checkmark next to or circle all that apply.

Date: **Day of Week**:   **Time**:   AM/PM

Reason for the session: Meal   Snack   Exercise   Other (Explain)

Meal Components: Protein   Fruit   Whole grain   Vegetable   Healthy Fat

Method of Preparation:

Baked	Broiled	Sautéed	Grilled	Boiled
Fried	Roasted	Steamed	Stir-fry	Stewed
Fresh/raw	Frozen	Canned	Processed/packaged	
Prepared by others	Other (Explain)			

Beverage Consumed:

Soda	Diet soda/seltzer water	Tap/bottled water
Milk/dairy alternative	Other (Explain)	

Exercise Location and Activity:

Level of Activity: Easy   Moderate   Vigorous   Highly Vigorous

Who joined you: **Or Circle:**   Ate Alone/Exercised Alone

Feelings experienced before/during/after and how you responded to those feelings? Were they expressed in the session? If so, how and if not, why not?

What positive step did you take or guardrail did you apply during this session? Did it go as planned? Would you do anything differently next time?

Activity Reflection

Journal some thoughts about the meal or snack you selected or the exercise you undertook. How did the meal/snack look, smell, and taste? What did you notice going on around you as you exercised? How were you in control of this session and how did this session control you?

Emotion Reflection

Journal about the feelings you experienced and how you responded to them. Was this session a reflection of feelings and emotions? List some positive self-talk responses you can offer to your internal critic to combat the lies you hear in your head.

When you complete your last session of Day 30, move on to the Phase Three Reflection.

**If you need more pages for Phase Three, you will find
an additional form to copy in the Appendix**

Phase Three Reflection

Congratulations on completing the third phase of your mindfulness journey! Now it is time to look back at where you have been over the last ten days. Look for small steps you took to apply guardrails that kept you from going over a cliff. Be honest regarding the places you didn't apply self-control and own the reasons why.

Take a few moments to honestly answer the following questions.

On average, how many times did you eat a meal or snack each day? What was the average time interval between them?

Was this different from Phase Two? How is it different? What led to the change? If it isn't any different, what prevented change?

On average, how many times did you exercise each day? What was the average duration of the session?

Was this different from Phase Two? How is it different? What led to the change? If it isn't any different, what prevented change?

Over the past ten days, did you see any changes in the focus of your sessions? If so, what led to the change? If not, what prevented a change? How did your focus change?

Who joined you most often or did you participate alone most often? How do you feel about that?

What did you notice most about your sessions related to your senses and awareness of your surroundings?

What are some guardrails you used? What are some guardrails you can use moving forward?

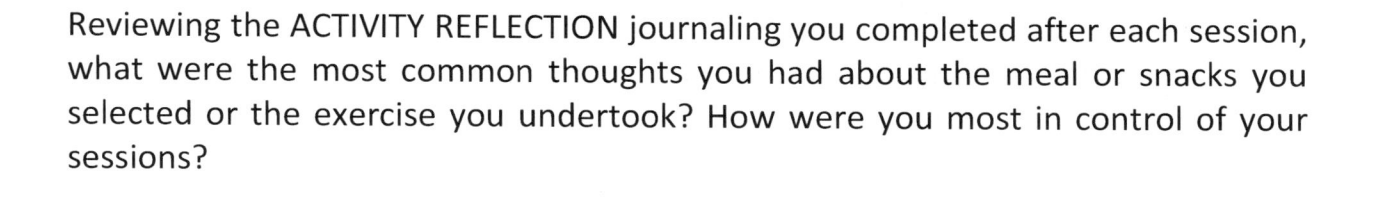

Reviewing the ACTIVITY REFLECTION journaling you completed after each session, what were the most common thoughts you had about the meal or snacks you selected or the exercise you undertook? How were you most in control of your sessions?

Reviewing the EMOTION REFLECTION journaling you completed after each session, how did you respond most often to feelings you experienced? Make a list of some of the best positive self-talk responses you came up with to combat negative thoughts from your internal critic.

How were your meals and snacks prepared most often over the last 10 days? Were you surprised by anything you learned about the meals and beverage patterns you saw? If so, what were they? If not, why were you not surprised?

Phase Four

Living a Nourishing and Active Life

You have come a long way over the last thirty days! Hopefully you can look back and see how far you have come. Now it is time to take the final steps forward in your mindfulness journey. During the next ten days you will begin focusing more attention on nourishing the body and being active for good health. This can be a hard ten days as you apply pressure to the chains of bondage and lean in with all your might to break them. Don't give up! Journal about the thoughts and feelings that come and recognize that a setback is just that, a step back. It doesn't mean you can't take a step forward again.

It is important to remember that we don't want to trade out old restrictive rules for new "healthy" rules. Trying to be "perfect" can become another form of bondage. Be mindful of behaviors, thoughts, and feelings that might be beginning to take you in that direction. We aren't looking to create new rules that put us in bondage. We do want to recognize healthy eating and exercise guidelines and begin to use those as the guidelines for the choices we make. At the same time, be mindful of your personal triggers as you take steps forward.

Here are some basic principles to help you build an eating plan that nourishes your body in a healthy way.

- The functions of the body are continuous 24 hours a day, seven days a week, 365 days a year. Nutrients are needed for the heart to pump, the muscles to move, and the nerve impulses to fire. Tissues need to be repaired, and hair and nails continue to grow. Be mindful about the nutrients you are giving to your body because it can only function well when it is fed well.
- It is best to eat several times a day using your satiety and hunger cues as a guide. Your metabolism or the rate at which your body will burn and use

the nutrients provided will set the pace. Select foods that are nutrient rich and that will nourish the body.

- The body needs water so it is important to consume water throughout the day. Usually eight to ten glasses is necessary to maintain proper hydration. Monitoring the color of your urine is an easy way to tell if you are adequately hydrated. Remember that caffeine dehydrates so the more caffeine you consume, the more water you will need to consume to compensate.
- Foods in whole form tend to be the most nutrient rich whether they are fresh or frozen. Take note of added sodium or sugars that can detract from the nutritional richness. Food labels that contain the least number of additives and preservatives usually are the most nutrient rich. Aim to limit pre-packed and processed foods as much as possible and consider whole foods that you could select in their place.
- Added sugar, salt, and fat decrease the nutritional richness of a food choice. Steaming, baking, broiling, or grilling is the healthiest method of food preparation and using seasonings and flavors that don't contain sodium or sugar is preferable.
- Try to select a lean protein and/or healthy fat source with a whole grain, fruit, and/or vegetable carbohydrate source at each meal and snack. This helps you feel satisfied longer and prevents large peaks and troughs in blood sugar levels that can bring about other impulsive responses. A hard boiled egg and an apple make a great mid-afternoon snack that can keep you satisfied until dinner.
- Recognize that all food groups provide important nutrients that are necessary for the body to function well. Omitting food groups for reasons other than a diagnosed medical condition can be unhealthy. All things are acceptable in moderation. There are no good and bad foods, only choices and selections that are best to make more often and choices and selections to be made less often. If you have medical reasons to limit or omit certain foods or food groups, work with your doctor or Registered Dietitian on a food plan that will work best for your individual needs.
- Meal planning doesn't have to be difficult and portion control doesn't have to control you. Here are some guidelines that can help you put it all together.
    - A nine to eleven inch plate is a good size to use for meals.

- Fill half of it with nutrient rich *vegetables*, prepared in a healthy way. Fresh is ideal but frozen is just as nutrient rich. Remember that many canned options contain additional sodium. Simply rinse before use and they still provide important nutrients to your plate.
  - Select a *lean protein source* that is prepared in a healthy way to fill one fourth of the other side.
  - Select a *whole grain* to fill the last quarter of the plate.
  - Select a *calcium source* as your beverage several times a day or include Greek yogurt or low fat cottage cheese along with your lean protein choice. If milk isn't something that agrees with you, select an unsweetened dairy alternative such as coconut, almond, or cashew milk.
  - Consider *fruit* as your dessert choice remembering that fresh fruits and berries are the most nutrient rich. Canned fruits packed in juice are also great options. Remember that fruits canned in syrup can be rinsed to make them a healthier choice as well.
- Be kind to yourself as you stretch and grow to find new foods and new ways to enjoy them. Be open to new things while also being mindful of your triggers. Build guardrails where needed so you can safely move around dangerous corners to new open roads.

It is important to find activities that you enjoy that don't focus on the calories used. Many people today have traded in the daily exercises of old. Instead of washing the car and push mowing the lawn, many of us use a car wash or riding mower. These activities get your body moving and your heart rate up while providing a sense of satisfaction once they are complete. Taking a dog or small child for a walk at the park or around the neighborhood can bring pleasure while also getting the heart pumping and blood circulating. Walking or jogging with a friend or training for a charity event that raises money for a cause you care about are new ways to change your focus. Strengthening your core and stretching can help with aches and pains you may be experiencing. Don't get hung up on numbers, sets, and length of time. Focus on how your body feels physically. Pay attention to your breathing patterns and your heart rate. Find joy in being active while not being in bondage to exercise.

The song "Put One Foot in Front of the Other" from the animated cartoon *Santa Claus is Coming to Town* depicts the process of change at its most basic; simply put one foot in front of the other. That's how you move forward. As the song says, "you'll never get where you're going, if you never get up on your feet…Put one foot in front of the other and soon you'll be walking across the floor."[1] Use these next ten days to get on your feet and get moving forward.

During these last ten days you will complete a session log for *each* food or exercise related activity you undertake, just as you did over the last thirty days. The focus this time will be on helping you evaluate the steps you are taking to incorporate a healthy and balanced eating and activity plan into your day to day life. Use all that you have learned over these last thirty days as you evaluate and journal about sessions.

Remember to use a *new entry* for each session. That is ideal, however, if you do not have the time to commit to that level of discovery, doing one entry at the end of the day that captures the highlights is also an option. If you run out of session journal entry space before your last session on day 40, please go to the appendix section of the journal and make additional copies. If you get to your last session of day 40 and you aren't at the end of the provided Phase Four journaling pages, move on to the Phase Four Reflection activity. Once you have completed your last session on day 40, take some time to complete the *Phase Four Reflection* questions.

Be sure to allow time to reflect and journal *after* each session as well as at the end of day 40.

---

1. Lyrics.com, STANDS4 LLC, 2019. "Put One Foot in Front of the Other [From Santa Claus Is Coming to Town] Lyrics." Accessed September 30, 2019. https://www.lyrics.com/lyric/1337724/Mickey+Rooney.

Phase Four Session Log Sheet

Day 31- Day 40

Complete the log for this food/exercise session. Place a checkmark next to or circle all that apply.

Date: **Day of Week**:   **Time**:   AM/PM

Reason for the session: Meal   Snack   Exercise   Other (Explain)

Meal Components: Protein   Fruit   Whole grain   Vegetable   Healthy Fat

Method of Preparation:

Baked	Broiled	Sautéed	Grilled	Boiled
Fried	Roasted	Steamed	Stir-fry	Stewed
Fresh/raw	Frozen	Canned	Processed/packaged	
Prepared by others	Other (Explain)			

Beverage Consumed:

Soda   Diet soda/seltzer water   Tap/bottled water
Milk/dairy alternative Other (Explain)

Exercise Location and Activity:

Level of Activity: Easy   Moderate   Vigorous   Highly Vigorous

Who joined you: **Or Circle**:   Ate Alone/Exercised Alone

Journal about the session. Did past behaviors, situations, or emotional responses impact the session? How was this a nourishing session to your body? What positive steps did you take?

When you complete your last session of Day 40, move on to the Phase Four Reflection.

Phase Four Session Log Sheet

Day 31- Day 40

Complete the log for this food/exercise session. Place a checkmark next to or circle all that apply.

Date:	**Day of Week:**	**Time:**	AM/PM

Reason for the session:	Meal	Snack	Exercise	Other (Explain)

Meal Components:	Protein	Fruit	Whole grain	Vegetable	Healthy Fat

Method of Preparation:

Baked	Broiled	Sautéed	Grilled	Boiled
Fried	Roasted	Steamed	Stir-fry	Stewed
Fresh/raw	Frozen	Canned	Processed/packaged	
Prepared by others	Other (Explain)			

Beverage Consumed:

Soda	Diet soda/seltzer water	Tap/bottled water
Milk/dairy alternative	Other (Explain)

Exercise Location and Activity:

Level of Activity:	Easy	Moderate	Vigorous	Highly Vigorous

Who joined you:	**Or Circle:**	Ate Alone/Exercised Alone

Journal about the session. Did past behaviors, situations, or emotional responses impact the session? How was this a nourishing session to your body? What positive steps did you take?

When you complete your last session of Day 40, move on to the Phase Four Reflection.

Phase Four Session Log Sheet

Day 31- Day 40

Complete the log for this food/exercise session. Place a checkmark next to or circle all that apply.

Date: **Day of Week**:   **Time**:   AM/PM

Reason for the session: Meal   Snack   Exercise   Other (Explain)

Meal Components: Protein   Fruit   Whole grain   Vegetable   Healthy Fat

Method of Preparation:

Baked	Broiled	Sautéed	Grilled	Boiled
Fried	Roasted	Steamed	Stir-fry	Stewed
Fresh/raw	Frozen	Canned	Processed/packaged	
Prepared by others	Other (Explain)			

Beverage Consumed:

Soda	Diet soda/seltzer water	Tap/bottled water
Milk/dairy alternative	Other (Explain)	

Exercise Location and Activity:

Level of Activity: Easy   Moderate   Vigorous   Highly Vigorous

Who joined you: **Or Circle**:   Ate Alone/Exercised Alone

Journal about the session. Did past behaviors, situations, or emotional responses impact the session? How was this a nourishing session to your body? What positive steps did you take?

When you complete your last session of Day 40, move on to the Phase Four Reflection.

Phase Four Session Log Sheet

Day 31- Day 40

Complete the log for this food/exercise session. Place a checkmark next to or circle all that apply.

Date: **Day of Week:** **Time:** AM/PM

Reason for the session: Meal Snack Exercise Other (Explain)

Meal Components: Protein Fruit Whole grain Vegetable Healthy Fat

Method of Preparation:

Baked	Broiled	Sautéed	Grilled	Boiled
Fried	Roasted	Steamed	Stir-fry	Stewed
Fresh/raw	Frozen	Canned	Processed/packaged	
Prepared by others	Other (Explain)			

Beverage Consumed:

Soda Diet soda/seltzer water Tap/bottled water
Milk/dairy alternative Other (Explain)

Exercise Location and Activity:

Level of Activity: Easy Moderate Vigorous Highly Vigorous

Who joined you: **Or Circle:** Ate Alone/Exercised Alone

Journal about the session. Did past behaviors, situations, or emotional responses impact the session? How was this a nourishing session to your body? What positive steps did you take?

When you complete your last session of Day 40, move on to the Phase Four Reflection.

Phase Four Session Log Sheet

Day 31- Day 40

Complete the log for this food/exercise session. Place a checkmark next to or circle all that apply.

Date: **Day of Week**:   **Time**:   AM/PM

Reason for the session: Meal   Snack   Exercise   Other (Explain)

Meal Components: Protein   Fruit   Whole grain   Vegetable   Healthy Fat

Method of Preparation:

Baked	Broiled	Sautéed	Grilled	Boiled
Fried	Roasted	Steamed	Stir-fry	Stewed
Fresh/raw	Frozen	Canned	Processed/packaged	
Prepared by others	Other (Explain)			

Beverage Consumed:

Soda   Diet soda/seltzer water   Tap/bottled water
Milk/dairy alternative   Other (Explain)

Exercise Location and Activity:

Level of Activity: Easy   Moderate   Vigorous   Highly Vigorous

Who joined you: **Or Circle**:   Ate Alone/Exercised Alone

Journal about the session. Did past behaviors, situations, or emotional responses impact the session? How was this a nourishing session to your body? What positive steps did you take?

When you complete your last session of Day 40, move on to the Phase Four Reflection.

Phase Four Session Log Sheet

Day 31- Day 40

Complete the log for this food/exercise session. Place a checkmark next to or circle all that apply.

Date: **Day of Week:** **Time:** AM/PM

Reason for the session: Meal Snack Exercise Other (Explain)

Meal Components: Protein Fruit Whole grain Vegetable Healthy Fat

Method of Preparation:

Baked	Broiled	Sautéed	Grilled	Boiled
Fried	Roasted	Steamed	Stir-fry	Stewed
Fresh/raw	Frozen	Canned	Processed/packaged	
Prepared by others	Other (Explain)			

Beverage Consumed:

Soda Diet soda/seltzer water Tap/bottled water
Milk/dairy alternative Other (Explain)

Exercise Location and Activity:

Level of Activity: Easy Moderate Vigorous Highly Vigorous

Who joined you: **Or Circle:** Ate Alone/Exercised Alone

Journal about the session. Did past behaviors, situations, or emotional responses impact the session? How was this a nourishing session to your body? What positive steps did you take?

When you complete your last session of Day 40, move on to the Phase Four Reflection.

Phase Four Session Log Sheet

Day 31- Day 40

Complete the log for this food/exercise session. Place a checkmark next to or circle all that apply.

Date:　　　　　　　　**Day of Week**:　　　　　　　　**Time**:　　　　　AM/PM

Reason for the session:　　Meal　　　　Snack　　　　Exercise　　　　Other (Explain)

Meal Components:　　Protein　　Fruit　　Whole grain　　Vegetable　　Healthy Fat

Method of Preparation:

Baked	Broiled	Sautéed	Grilled	Boiled
Fried	Roasted	Steamed	Stir-fry	Stewed
Fresh/raw	Frozen	Canned	Processed/packaged	
Prepared by others	Other (Explain)			

Beverage Consumed:

Soda	Diet soda/seltzer water	Tap/bottled water
Milk/dairy alternative	Other (Explain)	

Exercise Location and Activity:

Level of Activity:　　　　Easy　　　　Moderate　　　　Vigorous　　　　Highly Vigorous

Who joined you:　　　　　　　　**Or Circle**:　　　　Ate Alone/Exercised Alone

Journal about the session. Did past behaviors, situations, or emotional responses impact the session? How was this a nourishing session to your body? What positive steps did you take?

When you complete your last session of Day 40, move on to the Phase Four Reflection.

Phase Four Session Log Sheet

Day 31- Day 40

Complete the log for this food/exercise session. Place a checkmark next to or circle all that apply.

Date:　　　　　　　　　**Day of Week:**　　　　　　　　**Time:**　　　　　AM/PM

Reason for the session:　　Meal　　　　Snack　　　　Exercise　　　　Other (Explain)

Meal Components:　　Protein　　Fruit　　Whole grain　　Vegetable　　Healthy Fat

Method of Preparation:

Baked	Broiled	Sautéed	Grilled	Boiled
Fried	Roasted	Steamed	Stir-fry	Stewed
Fresh/raw	Frozen	Canned	Processed/packaged	
Prepared by others	Other (Explain)			

Beverage Consumed:

Soda　　　　　　　　　Diet soda/seltzer water　　　　Tap/bottled water
Milk/dairy alternative　Other (Explain)

Exercise Location and Activity:

Level of Activity:　　　Easy　　　　Moderate　　　　Vigorous　　　　Highly Vigorous

Who joined you:　　　　　　　　　　**Or Circle:**　　　Ate Alone/Exercised Alone

Journal about the session. Did past behaviors, situations, or emotional responses impact the session? How was this a nourishing session to your body? What positive steps did you take?

When you complete your last session of Day 40, move on to the Phase Four Reflection.

Phase Four Session Log Sheet

Day 31- Day 40

Complete the log for this food/exercise session. Place a checkmark next to or circle all that apply.

Date: **Day of Week**:   **Time**:   AM/PM

Reason for the session: Meal   Snack   Exercise   Other (Explain)

Meal Components: Protein   Fruit   Whole grain   Vegetable   Healthy Fat

Method of Preparation:

Baked	Broiled	Sautéed	Grilled	Boiled
Fried	Roasted	Steamed	Stir-fry	Stewed
Fresh/raw	Frozen	Canned	Processed/packaged	
Prepared by others	Other (Explain)			

Beverage Consumed:

Soda	Diet soda/seltzer water	Tap/bottled water
Milk/dairy alternative	Other (Explain)	

Exercise Location and Activity:

Level of Activity: Easy   Moderate   Vigorous   Highly Vigorous

Who joined you: **Or Circle**:   Ate Alone/Exercised Alone

Journal about the session. Did past behaviors, situations, or emotional responses impact the session? How was this a nourishing session to your body? What positive steps did you take?

When you complete your last session of Day 40, move on to the Phase Four Reflection.

Phase Four Session Log Sheet

Day 31- Day 40

Complete the log for this food/exercise session. Place a checkmark next to or circle all that apply.

Date: **Day of Week:**   **Time:**   AM/PM

Reason for the session: Meal   Snack   Exercise   Other (Explain)

Meal Components: Protein   Fruit   Whole grain   Vegetable   Healthy Fat

Method of Preparation:

Baked	Broiled	Sautéed	Grilled	Boiled
Fried	Roasted	Steamed	Stir-fry	Stewed
Fresh/raw	Frozen	Canned	Processed/packaged	
Prepared by others	Other (Explain)			

Beverage Consumed:

Soda   Diet soda/seltzer water   Tap/bottled water
Milk/dairy alternative   Other (Explain)

Exercise Location and Activity:

Level of Activity: Easy   Moderate   Vigorous   Highly Vigorous

Who joined you: **Or Circle:**   Ate Alone/Exercised Alone

Journal about the session. Did past behaviors, situations, or emotional responses impact the session? How was this a nourishing session to your body? What positive steps did you take?

When you complete your last session of Day 40, move on to the Phase Four Reflection.

Phase Four Session Log Sheet

Day 31- Day 40

Complete the log for this food/exercise session. Place a checkmark next to or circle all that apply.

Date: **Day of Week:** **Time:** AM/PM

Reason for the session: Meal Snack Exercise Other (Explain)

Meal Components: Protein Fruit Whole grain Vegetable Healthy Fat

Method of Preparation:

Baked	Broiled	Sautéed	Grilled	Boiled
Fried	Roasted	Steamed	Stir-fry	Stewed
Fresh/raw	Frozen	Canned	Processed/packaged	
Prepared by others	Other (Explain)			

Beverage Consumed:

Soda	Diet soda/seltzer water	Tap/bottled water
Milk/dairy alternative	Other (Explain)	

Exercise Location and Activity:

Level of Activity: Easy Moderate Vigorous Highly Vigorous

Who joined you: **Or Circle:** Ate Alone/Exercised Alone

Journal about the session. Did past behaviors, situations, or emotional responses impact the session? How was this a nourishing session to your body? What positive steps did you take?

When you complete your last session of Day 40, move on to the Phase Four Reflection.

Phase Four Session Log Sheet

Day 31- Day 40

Complete the log for this food/exercise session. Place a checkmark next to or circle all that apply.

Date: **Day of Week:**   **Time:**   AM/PM

Reason for the session: Meal   Snack   Exercise   Other (Explain)

Meal Components: Protein   Fruit   Whole grain   Vegetable   Healthy Fat

Method of Preparation:

Baked	Broiled	Sautéed	Grilled	Boiled
Fried	Roasted	Steamed	Stir-fry	Stewed
Fresh/raw	Frozen	Canned	Processed/packaged	
Prepared by others	Other (Explain)			

Beverage Consumed:

Soda	Diet soda/seltzer water	Tap/bottled water
Milk/dairy alternative	Other (Explain)	

Exercise Location and Activity:

Level of Activity: Easy   Moderate   Vigorous   Highly Vigorous

Who joined you: **Or Circle:**   Ate Alone/Exercised Alone

Journal about the session. Did past behaviors, situations, or emotional responses impact the session? How was this a nourishing session to your body? What positive steps did you take?

When you complete your last session of Day 40, move on to the Phase Four Reflection.

Phase Four Session Log Sheet

Day 31- Day 40

Complete the log for this food/exercise session. Place a checkmark next to or circle all that apply.

Date: **Day of Week:** **Time:** AM/PM

Reason for the session: Meal Snack Exercise Other (Explain)

Meal Components: Protein Fruit Whole grain Vegetable Healthy Fat

Method of Preparation:

Baked	Broiled	Sautéed	Grilled	Boiled
Fried	Roasted	Steamed	Stir-fry	Stewed
Fresh/raw	Frozen	Canned	Processed/packaged	
Prepared by others	Other (Explain)			

Beverage Consumed:

Soda	Diet soda/seltzer water	Tap/bottled water
Milk/dairy alternative	Other (Explain)	

Exercise Location and Activity:

Level of Activity: Easy Moderate Vigorous Highly Vigorous

Who joined you: **Or Circle:** Ate Alone/Exercised Alone

Journal about the session. Did past behaviors, situations, or emotional responses impact the session? How was this a nourishing session to your body? What positive steps did you take?

When you complete your last session of Day 40, move on to the Phase Four Reflection.

Phase Four Session Log Sheet

Day 31- Day 40

Complete the log for this food/exercise session. Place a checkmark next to or circle all that apply.

Date: **Day of Week:**   **Time:**   AM/PM

Reason for the session: Meal   Snack   Exercise   Other (Explain)

Meal Components: Protein   Fruit   Whole grain   Vegetable   Healthy Fat

Method of Preparation:

Baked	Broiled	Sautéed	Grilled	Boiled
Fried	Roasted	Steamed	Stir-fry	Stewed
Fresh/raw	Frozen	Canned	Processed/packaged	
Prepared by others	Other (Explain)			

Beverage Consumed:

Soda   Diet soda/seltzer water   Tap/bottled water
Milk/dairy alternative Other (Explain)

Exercise Location and Activity:

Level of Activity: Easy   Moderate   Vigorous   Highly Vigorous

Who joined you: **Or Circle:**   Ate Alone/Exercised Alone

Journal about the session. Did past behaviors, situations, or emotional responses impact the session? How was this a nourishing session to your body? What positive steps did you take?

When you complete your last session of Day 40, move on to the Phase Four Reflection.

Phase Four Session Log Sheet

Day 31- Day 40

Complete the log for this food/exercise session. Place a checkmark next to or circle all that apply.

Date:　　　　　　　　**Day of Week**:　　　　　　　　**Time**:　　　　AM/PM

Reason for the session:　　Meal　　　　Snack　　　　Exercise　　　　Other (Explain)

Meal Components:　　Protein　　Fruit　　Whole grain　　Vegetable　　Healthy Fat

Method of Preparation:

Baked	Broiled	Sautéed	Grilled	Boiled
Fried	Roasted	Steamed	Stir-fry	Stewed
Fresh/raw	Frozen	Canned	Processed/packaged	
Prepared by others	Other (Explain)			

Beverage Consumed:

Soda	Diet soda/seltzer water	Tap/bottled water
Milk/dairy alternative	Other (Explain)	

Exercise Location and Activity:

Level of Activity:　　　　Easy　　　　Moderate　　　　Vigorous　　　　Highly Vigorous

Who joined you:　　　　　　　　**Or Circle**:　　　　Ate Alone/Exercised Alone

Journal about the session. Did past behaviors, situations, or emotional responses impact the session? How was this a nourishing session to your body? What positive steps did you take?

When you complete your last session of Day 40, move on to the Phase Four Reflection.

Phase Four Session Log Sheet

Day 31- Day 40

Complete the log for this food/exercise session. Place a checkmark next to or circle all that apply.

Date:　　　　　　　**Day of Week:**　　　　　　　**Time:**　　　　　AM/PM

Reason for the session:　　Meal　　　　Snack　　　　Exercise　　　　Other (Explain)

Meal Components:　　Protein　　Fruit　　Whole grain　　Vegetable　　Healthy Fat

Method of Preparation:

Baked	Broiled	Sautéed	Grilled	Boiled
Fried	Roasted	Steamed	Stir-fry	Stewed
Fresh/raw	Frozen	Canned	Processed/packaged	
Prepared by others	Other (Explain)			

Beverage Consumed:

Soda	Diet soda/seltzer water	Tap/bottled water
Milk/dairy alternative	Other (Explain)	

Exercise Location and Activity:

Level of Activity:　　　Easy　　　　Moderate　　　　Vigorous　　　　Highly Vigorous

Who joined you:　　　　　　　**Or Circle:**　　　　Ate Alone/Exercised Alone

Journal about the session. Did past behaviors, situations, or emotional responses impact the session? How was this a nourishing session to your body? What positive steps did you take?

When you complete your last session of Day 40, move on to the Phase Four Reflection.

Phase Four Session Log Sheet

Day 31- Day 40

Complete the log for this food/exercise session. Place a checkmark next to or circle all that apply.

Date: **Day of Week**: **Time**: AM/PM

Reason for the session: Meal   Snack   Exercise   Other (Explain)

Meal Components: Protein   Fruit   Whole grain   Vegetable   Healthy Fat

Method of Preparation:

Baked	Broiled	Sautéed	Grilled	Boiled
Fried	Roasted	Steamed	Stir-fry	Stewed
Fresh/raw	Frozen	Canned	Processed/packaged	
Prepared by others	Other (Explain)			

Beverage Consumed:

Soda	Diet soda/seltzer water	Tap/bottled water
Milk/dairy alternative	Other (Explain)	

Exercise Location and Activity:

Level of Activity: Easy   Moderate   Vigorous   Highly Vigorous

Who joined you: **Or Circle**:   Ate Alone/Exercised Alone

Journal about the session. Did past behaviors, situations, or emotional responses impact the session? How was this a nourishing session to your body? What positive steps did you take?

When you complete your last session of Day 40, move on to the Phase Four Reflection.

Phase Four Session Log Sheet

Day 31- Day 40

Complete the log for this food/exercise session. Place a checkmark next to or circle all that apply.

Date:　　　　　　　**Day of Week:**　　　　　　　**Time:**　　　　AM/PM

Reason for the session:　　Meal　　　　Snack　　　　Exercise　　　　Other (Explain)

Meal Components:　　Protein　　Fruit　　Whole grain　　Vegetable　　Healthy Fat

Method of Preparation:

Baked	Broiled	Sautéed	Grilled	Boiled
Fried	Roasted	Steamed	Stir-fry	Stewed
Fresh/raw	Frozen	Canned	Processed/packaged	
Prepared by others	Other (Explain)			

Beverage Consumed:

Soda	Diet soda/seltzer water	Tap/bottled water
Milk/dairy alternative	Other (Explain)	

Exercise Location and Activity:

Level of Activity:　　　　Easy　　　　Moderate　　　　Vigorous　　　　Highly Vigorous

Who joined you:　　　　　　　　**Or Circle:**　　　Ate Alone/Exercised Alone

Journal about the session. Did past behaviors, situations, or emotional responses impact the session? How was this a nourishing session to your body? What positive steps did you take?

When you complete your last session of Day 40, move on to the Phase Four Reflection.

Phase Four Session Log Sheet

Day 31- Day 40

Complete the log for this food/exercise session. Place a checkmark next to or circle all that apply.

Date:　　　　　　　　　**Day of Week:**　　　　　　　　**Time:**　　　　　AM/PM

Reason for the session:　　Meal　　　　Snack　　　　Exercise　　　　Other (Explain)

Meal Components:　　Protein　　Fruit　　Whole grain　　Vegetable　　Healthy Fat

Method of Preparation:

Baked	Broiled	Sautéed	Grilled	Boiled
Fried	Roasted	Steamed	Stir-fry	Stewed
Fresh/raw	Frozen	Canned	Processed/packaged	
Prepared by others	Other (Explain)			

Beverage Consumed:

Soda	Diet soda/seltzer water	Tap/bottled water
Milk/dairy alternative	Other (Explain)	

Exercise Location and Activity:

Level of Activity:　　　　Easy　　　　Moderate　　　　Vigorous　　　　Highly Vigorous

Who joined you:　　　　　　　　**Or Circle:**　　　　Ate Alone/Exercised Alone

Journal about the session. Did past behaviors, situations, or emotional responses impact the session? How was this a nourishing session to your body? What positive steps did you take?

When you complete your last session of Day 40, move on to the Phase Four Reflection.

Phase Four Session Log Sheet

Day 31- Day 40

Complete the log for this food/exercise session. Place a checkmark next to or circle all that apply.

Date: **Day of Week:** **Time:** AM/PM

Reason for the session: Meal Snack Exercise Other (Explain)

Meal Components: Protein Fruit Whole grain Vegetable Healthy Fat

Method of Preparation:

Baked	Broiled	Sautéed	Grilled	Boiled
Fried	Roasted	Steamed	Stir-fry	Stewed
Fresh/raw	Frozen	Canned	Processed/packaged	
Prepared by others	Other (Explain)			

Beverage Consumed:

Soda Diet soda/seltzer water Tap/bottled water
Milk/dairy alternative Other (Explain)

Exercise Location and Activity:

Level of Activity: Easy Moderate Vigorous Highly Vigorous

Who joined you: **Or Circle:** Ate Alone/Exercised Alone

Journal about the session. Did past behaviors, situations, or emotional responses impact the session? How was this a nourishing session to your body? What positive steps did you take?

When you complete your last session of Day 40, move on to the Phase Four Reflection.

Phase Four Session Log Sheet

Day 31- Day 40

Complete the log for this food/exercise session. Place a checkmark next to or circle all that apply.

Date: **Day of Week:**   **Time:**   AM/PM

Reason for the session: Meal   Snack   Exercise   Other (Explain)

Meal Components: Protein   Fruit   Whole grain   Vegetable   Healthy Fat

Method of Preparation:

Baked	Broiled	Sautéed	Grilled	Boiled
Fried	Roasted	Steamed	Stir-fry	Stewed
Fresh/raw	Frozen	Canned	Processed/packaged	
Prepared by others	Other (Explain)			

Beverage Consumed:

Soda	Diet soda/seltzer water	Tap/bottled water
Milk/dairy alternative	Other (Explain)	

Exercise Location and Activity:

Level of Activity: Easy   Moderate   Vigorous   Highly Vigorous

Who joined you: **Or Circle:**   Ate Alone/Exercised Alone

Journal about the session. Did past behaviors, situations, or emotional responses impact the session? How was this a nourishing session to your body? What positive steps did you take?

When you complete your last session of Day 40, move on to the Phase Four Reflection.

Phase Four Session Log Sheet

Day 31- Day 40

Complete the log for this food/exercise session. Place a checkmark next to or circle all that apply.

Date:　　　　　　　　**Day of Week:**　　　　　　　　**Time:**　　　　AM/PM

Reason for the session:　　Meal　　　　Snack　　　　Exercise　　　　Other (Explain)

Meal Components:　　Protein　　Fruit　　Whole grain　　Vegetable　　Healthy Fat

Method of Preparation:

Baked	Broiled	Sautéed	Grilled	Boiled
Fried	Roasted	Steamed	Stir-fry	Stewed
Fresh/raw	Frozen	Canned	Processed/packaged	
Prepared by others	Other (Explain)			

Beverage Consumed:

Soda	Diet soda/seltzer water	Tap/bottled water
Milk/dairy alternative	Other (Explain)	

Exercise Location and Activity:

Level of Activity:　　　　Easy　　　　Moderate　　　　Vigorous　　　　Highly Vigorous

Who joined you:　　　　　　　　　　**Or Circle:**　　　　Ate Alone/Exercised Alone

Journal about the session. Did past behaviors, situations, or emotional responses impact the session? How was this a nourishing session to your body? What positive steps did you take?

When you complete your last session of Day 40, move on to the Phase Four Reflection.

Phase Four Session Log Sheet

Day 31- Day 40

Complete the log for this food/exercise session. Place a checkmark next to or circle all that apply.

Date: **Day of Week**: **Time**: AM/PM

Reason for the session: Meal   Snack   Exercise   Other (Explain)

Meal Components: Protein   Fruit   Whole grain   Vegetable   Healthy Fat

Method of Preparation:

Baked	Broiled	Sautéed	Grilled	Boiled
Fried	Roasted	Steamed	Stir-fry	Stewed
Fresh/raw	Frozen	Canned	Processed/packaged	
Prepared by others	Other (Explain)			

Beverage Consumed:

Soda   Diet soda/seltzer water   Tap/bottled water
Milk/dairy alternative   Other (Explain)

Exercise Location and Activity:

Level of Activity: Easy   Moderate   Vigorous   Highly Vigorous

Who joined you: **Or Circle**:   Ate Alone/Exercised Alone

Journal about the session. Did past behaviors, situations, or emotional responses impact the session? How was this a nourishing session to your body? What positive steps did you take?

When you complete your last session of Day 40, move on to the Phase Four Reflection.

Phase Four Session Log Sheet

Day 31- Day 40

Complete the log for this food/exercise session. Place a checkmark next to or circle all that apply.

Date: **Day of Week:** **Time:** AM/PM

Reason for the session: Meal   Snack   Exercise   Other (Explain)

Meal Components: Protein   Fruit   Whole grain   Vegetable   Healthy Fat

Method of Preparation:

Baked	Broiled	Sautéed	Grilled	Boiled
Fried	Roasted	Steamed	Stir-fry	Stewed
Fresh/raw	Frozen	Canned	Processed/packaged	
Prepared by others	Other (Explain)			

Beverage Consumed:

Soda	Diet soda/seltzer water	Tap/bottled water
Milk/dairy alternative	Other (Explain)	

Exercise Location and Activity:

Level of Activity: Easy   Moderate   Vigorous   Highly Vigorous

Who joined you: **Or Circle:**   Ate Alone/Exercised Alone

Journal about the session. Did past behaviors, situations, or emotional responses impact the session? How was this a nourishing session to your body? What positive steps did you take?

When you complete your last session of Day 40, move on to the Phase Four Reflection.

Phase Four Session Log Sheet

Day 31- Day 40

Complete the log for this food/exercise session. Place a checkmark next to or circle all that apply.

Date:　　　　　　　　**Day of Week:**　　　　　　　　**Time:**　　　　　AM/PM

Reason for the session:　　Meal　　　　Snack　　　　Exercise　　　　Other (Explain)

Meal Components:　　Protein　　Fruit　　Whole grain　　Vegetable　　Healthy Fat

Method of Preparation:

Baked	Broiled	Sautéed	Grilled	Boiled
Fried	Roasted	Steamed	Stir-fry	Stewed
Fresh/raw	Frozen	Canned	Processed/packaged	
Prepared by others	Other (Explain)			

Beverage Consumed:

Soda	Diet soda/seltzer water	Tap/bottled water
Milk/dairy alternative	Other (Explain)	

Exercise Location and Activity:

Level of Activity:　　　　Easy　　　　Moderate　　　　Vigorous　　　　Highly Vigorous

Who joined you:　　　　　　　　**Or Circle:**　　　　Ate Alone/Exercised Alone

Journal about the session. Did past behaviors, situations, or emotional responses impact the session? How was this a nourishing session to your body? What positive steps did you take?

When you complete your last session of Day 40, move on to the Phase Four Reflection.

Phase Four Session Log Sheet

Day 31- Day 40

Complete the log for this food/exercise session. Place a checkmark next to or circle all that apply.

Date: **Day of Week**: **Time**: AM/PM

Reason for the session: Meal Snack Exercise Other (Explain)

Meal Components: Protein Fruit Whole grain Vegetable Healthy Fat

Method of Preparation:

Baked	Broiled	Sautéed	Grilled	Boiled
Fried	Roasted	Steamed	Stir-fry	Stewed
Fresh/raw	Frozen	Canned	Processed/packaged	
Prepared by others	Other (Explain)			

Beverage Consumed:

Soda Diet soda/seltzer water Tap/bottled water
Milk/dairy alternative Other (Explain)

Exercise Location and Activity:

Level of Activity: Easy Moderate Vigorous Highly Vigorous

Who joined you: **Or Circle**: Ate Alone/Exercised Alone

Journal about the session. Did past behaviors, situations, or emotional responses impact the session? How was this a nourishing session to your body? What positive steps did you take?

When you complete your last session of Day 40, move on to the Phase Four Reflection.

Phase Four Session Log Sheet

Day 31- Day 40

Complete the log for this food/exercise session. Place a checkmark next to or circle all that apply.

Date:　　　　　　　　**Day of Week**:　　　　　　　　**Time**:　　　　　AM/PM

Reason for the session:　　Meal　　　　Snack　　　　Exercise　　　　Other (Explain)

Meal Components:　　Protein　　Fruit　　Whole grain　　Vegetable　　Healthy Fat

Method of Preparation:

Baked	Broiled	Sautéed	Grilled	Boiled
Fried	Roasted	Steamed	Stir-fry	Stewed
Fresh/raw	Frozen	Canned	Processed/packaged	
Prepared by others	Other (Explain)			

Beverage Consumed:

Soda	Diet soda/seltzer water	Tap/bottled water
Milk/dairy alternative	Other (Explain)	

Exercise Location and Activity:

Level of Activity:　　　Easy　　　　Moderate　　　　Vigorous　　　　Highly Vigorous

Who joined you:　　　　　　　　**Or Circle**:　　　　Ate Alone/Exercised Alone

Journal about the session. Did past behaviors, situations, or emotional responses impact the session? How was this a nourishing session to your body? What positive steps did you take?

When you complete your last session of Day 40, move on to the Phase Four Reflection.

Phase Four Session Log Sheet

Day 31- Day 40

Complete the log for this food/exercise session. Place a checkmark next to or circle all that apply.

Date:　　　　　　　　　**Day of Week:**　　　　　　　　**Time:**　　　　AM/PM

Reason for the session:　　Meal　　　　Snack　　　　Exercise　　　　Other (Explain)

Meal Components:　　Protein　　Fruit　　Whole grain　　Vegetable　　Healthy Fat

Method of Preparation:

Baked	Broiled	Sautéed	Grilled	Boiled
Fried	Roasted	Steamed	Stir-fry	Stewed
Fresh/raw	Frozen	Canned	Processed/packaged	
Prepared by others	Other (Explain)			

Beverage Consumed:

Soda	Diet soda/seltzer water	Tap/bottled water
Milk/dairy alternative	Other (Explain)	

Exercise Location and Activity:

Level of Activity:　　　　Easy　　　　Moderate　　　　Vigorous　　　　Highly Vigorous

Who joined you:　　　　　　　　　　**Or Circle:**　　　Ate Alone/Exercised Alone

Journal about the session. Did past behaviors, situations, or emotional responses impact the session? How was this a nourishing session to your body? What positive steps did you take?

When you complete your last session of Day 40, move on to the Phase Four Reflection.

Phase Four Session Log Sheet

Day 31- Day 40

Complete the log for this food/exercise session. Place a checkmark next to or circle all that apply.

Date: **Day of Week:**   **Time:**   AM/PM

Reason for the session: Meal   Snack   Exercise   Other (Explain)

Meal Components: Protein   Fruit   Whole grain   Vegetable   Healthy Fat

Method of Preparation:

Baked	Broiled	Sautéed	Grilled	Boiled
Fried	Roasted	Steamed	Stir-fry	Stewed
Fresh/raw	Frozen	Canned	Processed/packaged	
Prepared by others	Other (Explain)			

Beverage Consumed:

Soda   Diet soda/seltzer water   Tap/bottled water
Milk/dairy alternative Other (Explain)

Exercise Location and Activity:

Level of Activity: Easy   Moderate   Vigorous   Highly Vigorous

Who joined you: **Or Circle:**   Ate Alone/Exercised Alone

Journal about the session. Did past behaviors, situations, or emotional responses impact the session? How was this a nourishing session to your body? What positive steps did you take?

When you complete your last session of Day 40, move on to the Phase Four Reflection.

Phase Four Session Log Sheet

Day 31- Day 40

Complete the log for this food/exercise session. Place a checkmark next to or circle all that apply.

Date: **Day of Week:**   **Time:**   AM/PM

Reason for the session: Meal   Snack   Exercise   Other (Explain)

Meal Components: Protein   Fruit   Whole grain   Vegetable   Healthy Fat

Method of Preparation:

Baked	Broiled	Sautéed	Grilled	Boiled
Fried	Roasted	Steamed	Stir-fry	Stewed
Fresh/raw	Frozen	Canned	Processed/packaged	
Prepared by others	Other (Explain)			

Beverage Consumed:

Soda	Diet soda/seltzer water	Tap/bottled water
Milk/dairy alternative	Other (Explain)	

Exercise Location and Activity:

Level of Activity: Easy   Moderate   Vigorous   Highly Vigorous

Who joined you: **Or Circle:**   Ate Alone/Exercised Alone

Journal about the session. Did past behaviors, situations, or emotional responses impact the session? How was this a nourishing session to your body? What positive steps did you take?

When you complete your last session of Day 40, move on to the Phase Four Reflection.

Phase Four Session Log Sheet

Day 31- Day 40

Complete the log for this food/exercise session. Place a checkmark next to or circle all that apply.

Date:　　　　　　　　**Day of Week:**　　　　　　　　**Time:**　　　　AM/PM

Reason for the session:　　Meal　　　　Snack　　　　Exercise　　　　Other (Explain)

Meal Components:　　Protein　　Fruit　　Whole grain　　Vegetable　　Healthy Fat

Method of Preparation:

Baked	Broiled	Sautéed	Grilled	Boiled
Fried	Roasted	Steamed	Stir-fry	Stewed
Fresh/raw	Frozen	Canned	Processed/packaged	
Prepared by others	Other (Explain)			

Beverage Consumed:

Soda	Diet soda/seltzer water	Tap/bottled water
Milk/dairy alternative	Other (Explain)	

Exercise Location and Activity:

Level of Activity:　　　　Easy　　　　Moderate　　　　Vigorous　　　　Highly Vigorous

Who joined you:　　　　　　　　**Or Circle:**　　　　Ate Alone/Exercised Alone

Journal about the session. Did past behaviors, situations, or emotional responses impact the session? How was this a nourishing session to your body? What positive steps did you take?

When you complete your last session of Day 40, move on to the Phase Four Reflection.

Phase Four Session Log Sheet

Day 31- Day 40

Complete the log for this food/exercise session. Place a checkmark next to or circle all that apply.

Date: **Day of Week:**   **Time:**   AM/PM

Reason for the session: Meal   Snack   Exercise   Other (Explain)

Meal Components: Protein   Fruit   Whole grain   Vegetable   Healthy Fat

Method of Preparation:

Baked	Broiled	Sautéed	Grilled	Boiled
Fried	Roasted	Steamed	Stir-fry	Stewed
Fresh/raw	Frozen	Canned	Processed/packaged	
Prepared by others	Other (Explain)			

Beverage Consumed:

Soda   Diet soda/seltzer water   Tap/bottled water
Milk/dairy alternative   Other (Explain)

Exercise Location and Activity:

Level of Activity: Easy   Moderate   Vigorous   Highly Vigorous

Who joined you: **Or Circle:**   Ate Alone/Exercised Alone

Journal about the session. Did past behaviors, situations, or emotional responses impact the session? How was this a nourishing session to your body? What positive steps did you take?

When you complete your last session of Day 40, move on to the Phase Four Reflection.

Phase Four Session Log Sheet

Day 31- Day 40

Complete the log for this food/exercise session. Place a checkmark next to or circle all that apply.

Date: **Day of Week:**   **Time:**   AM/PM

Reason for the session: Meal   Snack   Exercise   Other (Explain)

Meal Components: Protein   Fruit   Whole grain   Vegetable   Healthy Fat

Method of Preparation:

Baked	Broiled	Sautéed	Grilled	Boiled
Fried	Roasted	Steamed	Stir-fry	Stewed
Fresh/raw	Frozen	Canned	Processed/packaged	
Prepared by others	Other (Explain)			

Beverage Consumed:

Soda	Diet soda/seltzer water	Tap/bottled water
Milk/dairy alternative	Other (Explain)	

Exercise Location and Activity:

Level of Activity: Easy   Moderate   Vigorous   Highly Vigorous

Who joined you: **Or Circle:**   Ate Alone/Exercised Alone

Journal about the session. Did past behaviors, situations, or emotional responses impact the session? How was this a nourishing session to your body? What positive steps did you take?

When you complete your last session of Day 40, move on to the Phase Four Reflection.

Phase Four Session Log Sheet

Day 31- Day 40

Complete the log for this food/exercise session. Place a checkmark next to or circle all that apply.

Date:　　　　　　　　**Day of Week:**　　　　　　　　**Time:**　　　　　AM/PM

Reason for the session:　　Meal　　　　Snack　　　　Exercise　　　　Other (Explain)

Meal Components:　　Protein　　Fruit　　Whole grain　　Vegetable　　Healthy Fat

Method of Preparation:

Baked	Broiled	Sautéed	Grilled	Boiled
Fried	Roasted	Steamed	Stir-fry	Stewed
Fresh/raw	Frozen	Canned	Processed/packaged	
Prepared by others	Other (Explain)			

Beverage Consumed:

Soda	Diet soda/seltzer water	Tap/bottled water
Milk/dairy alternative	Other (Explain)	

Exercise Location and Activity:

Level of Activity:　　　　Easy　　　　Moderate　　　　Vigorous　　　　Highly Vigorous

Who joined you:　　　　　　　　**Or Circle:**　　　　Ate Alone/Exercised Alone

Journal about the session. Did past behaviors, situations, or emotional responses impact the session? How was this a nourishing session to your body? What positive steps did you take?

When you complete your last session of Day 40, move on to the Phase Four Reflection.

Phase Four Session Log Sheet

Day 31- Day 40

Complete the log for this food/exercise session. Place a checkmark next to or circle all that apply.

Date:　　　　　　　　　　**Day of Week:**　　　　　　　　**Time:**　　　　　　AM/PM

Reason for the session:　　Meal　　　　Snack　　　　Exercise　　　　Other (Explain)

Meal Components:　　Protein　　Fruit　　Whole grain　　Vegetable　　Healthy Fat

Method of Preparation:

Baked	Broiled	Sautéed	Grilled	Boiled
Fried	Roasted	Steamed	Stir-fry	Stewed
Fresh/raw	Frozen	Canned	Processed/packaged	
Prepared by others	Other (Explain)			

Beverage Consumed:

Soda　　　　　　　　　　Diet soda/seltzer water　　　　　Tap/bottled water
Milk/dairy alternative　　Other (Explain)

Exercise Location and Activity:

Level of Activity:　　　　Easy　　　　Moderate　　　　Vigorous　　　　Highly Vigorous

Who joined you:　　　　　　　　　　**Or Circle:**　　　　Ate Alone/Exercised Alone

Journal about the session. Did past behaviors, situations, or emotional responses impact the session? How was this a nourishing session to your body? What positive steps did you take?

When you complete your last session of Day 40, move on to the Phase Four Reflection.

Phase Four Session Log Sheet

Day 31- Day 40

Complete the log for this food/exercise session. Place a checkmark next to or circle all that apply.

Date: **Day of Week:** **Time:** AM/PM

Reason for the session: Meal Snack Exercise Other (Explain)

Meal Components: Protein Fruit Whole grain Vegetable Healthy Fat

Method of Preparation:

Baked	Broiled	Sautéed	Grilled	Boiled
Fried	Roasted	Steamed	Stir-fry	Stewed
Fresh/raw	Frozen	Canned	Processed/packaged	
Prepared by others	Other (Explain)			

Beverage Consumed:

Soda Diet soda/seltzer water Tap/bottled water
Milk/dairy alternative Other (Explain)

Exercise Location and Activity:

Level of Activity: Easy Moderate Vigorous Highly Vigorous

Who joined you: **Or Circle:** Ate Alone/Exercised Alone

Journal about the session. Did past behaviors, situations, or emotional responses impact the session? How was this a nourishing session to your body? What positive steps did you take?

When you complete your last session of Day 40, move on to the Phase Four Reflection.

Phase Four Session Log Sheet

Day 31- Day 40

Complete the log for this food/exercise session. Place a checkmark next to or circle all that apply.

Date: **Day of Week:** **Time:** AM/PM

Reason for the session: Meal   Snack   Exercise   Other (Explain)

Meal Components: Protein   Fruit   Whole grain   Vegetable   Healthy Fat

Method of Preparation:

Baked	Broiled	Sautéed	Grilled	Boiled
Fried	Roasted	Steamed	Stir-fry	Stewed
Fresh/raw	Frozen	Canned	Processed/packaged	
Prepared by others	Other (Explain)			

Beverage Consumed:

Soda	Diet soda/seltzer water	Tap/bottled water
Milk/dairy alternative	Other (Explain)	

Exercise Location and Activity:

Level of Activity: Easy   Moderate   Vigorous   Highly Vigorous

Who joined you: **Or Circle:**   Ate Alone/Exercised Alone

Journal about the session. Did past behaviors, situations, or emotional responses impact the session? How was this a nourishing session to your body? What positive steps did you take?

When you complete your last session of Day 40, move on to the Phase Four Reflection.

Phase Four Session Log Sheet

Day 31- Day 40

Complete the log for this food/exercise session. Place a checkmark next to or circle all that apply.

Date: **Day of Week:** **Time:** AM/PM

Reason for the session: Meal Snack Exercise Other (Explain)

Meal Components: Protein Fruit Whole grain Vegetable Healthy Fat

Method of Preparation:

Baked	Broiled	Sautéed	Grilled	Boiled
Fried	Roasted	Steamed	Stir-fry	Stewed
Fresh/raw	Frozen	Canned	Processed/packaged	
Prepared by others	Other (Explain)			

Beverage Consumed:

Soda Diet soda/seltzer water Tap/bottled water
Milk/dairy alternative Other (Explain)

Exercise Location and Activity:

Level of Activity: Easy Moderate Vigorous Highly Vigorous

Who joined you: **Or Circle:** Ate Alone/Exercised Alone

Journal about the session. Did past behaviors, situations, or emotional responses impact the session? How was this a nourishing session to your body? What positive steps did you take?

When you complete your last session of Day 40, move on to the Phase Four Reflection.

Phase Four Session Log Sheet

Day 31- Day 40

Complete the log for this food/exercise session. Place a checkmark next to or circle all that apply.

Date: **Day of Week**: **Time**: AM/PM

Reason for the session: Meal   Snack   Exercise   Other (Explain)

Meal Components: Protein   Fruit   Whole grain   Vegetable   Healthy Fat

Method of Preparation:

Baked	Broiled	Sautéed	Grilled	Boiled
Fried	Roasted	Steamed	Stir-fry	Stewed
Fresh/raw	Frozen	Canned	Processed/packaged	
Prepared by others	Other (Explain)			

Beverage Consumed:

Soda   Diet soda/seltzer water   Tap/bottled water
Milk/dairy alternative   Other (Explain)

Exercise Location and Activity:

Level of Activity: Easy   Moderate   Vigorous   Highly Vigorous

Who joined you: **Or Circle**:   Ate Alone/Exercised Alone

Journal about the session. Did past behaviors, situations, or emotional responses impact the session? How was this a nourishing session to your body? What positive steps did you take?

When you complete your last session of Day 40, move on to the Phase Four Reflection.

Phase Four Session Log Sheet

Day 31- Day 40

Complete the log for this food/exercise session. Place a checkmark next to or circle all that apply.

Date: **Day of Week:** **Time:** AM/PM

Reason for the session: Meal Snack Exercise Other (Explain)

Meal Components: Protein Fruit Whole grain Vegetable Healthy Fat

Method of Preparation:

Baked	Broiled	Sautéed	Grilled	Boiled
Fried	Roasted	Steamed	Stir-fry	Stewed
Fresh/raw	Frozen	Canned	Processed/packaged	
Prepared by others	Other (Explain)			

Beverage Consumed:

Soda	Diet soda/seltzer water	Tap/bottled water
Milk/dairy alternative	Other (Explain)	

Exercise Location and Activity:

Level of Activity: Easy Moderate Vigorous Highly Vigorous

Who joined you: **Or Circle:** Ate Alone/Exercised Alone

Journal about the session. Did past behaviors, situations, or emotional responses impact the session? How was this a nourishing session to your body? What positive steps did you take?

When you complete your last session of Day 40, move on to the Phase Four Reflection.

If you need more pages for Phase Four, you will find an additional form to copy in the Appendix

Phase Four Reflection

Congratulations on completing the final phase of your mindfulness journey! Now it is time to look back at where you have been over the last ten days. Look for small steps you took to nourish your body and apply all that you have discovered over the last 40 days.

Take a few moments to honestly answer the following questions.

On average, how many times did you eat a meal or snack each day? What was the average time interval between them?

What did most of your meals and snacks consist of and what method of preparation was selected most often?

Journal about how this new pattern was different from your patterns in Phase One and how the changes reflect your mindfulness journey.

On average, how many times did you exercise each day? How many times did you exercise over the previous ten days? What was the average duration of the session?

Journal about how this new pattern was different from your patterns in Phase One and how the changes reflect your mindfulness journey.

What did you notice about your sessions related to behaviors, situations, or emotional responses?

Journal about the changes you notice from those experienced at the end of Phase One.

Journal about the positive steps forward you have taken to nourish your body through food and activity during these last ten days.

Looking back at Phase One and your previous eating and exercise practices compared to today, write a list of affirmative statements to yourself about all the positive steps you have made over the last 40 days.

Wrapping Up

Congratulations on completing your mindfulness journey! Hopefully you can see many ways you have created a healthier relationship with food and exercise. Those results came because of the time and effort you put in over the last forty days. Now that you have broken the strongholds, your journey doesn't end. This is just the beginning!

Take a few moments to think about these questions. Who told us that we weren't supposed to gain weight or have changes in our bodies as we age? Is it realistic to think a 12-year-old and a 32-year-old person should be the same weight and look the same? If not, then why should a 32-year- old and a 52-year-old person weigh or look the same? Where did the idea come from that everyone should be the same shape and size? If we are not all genetically identical, why would we expect to be the same size and shape as someone else? Are we creating the healthiest and best version of ourselves inside and out? Or, are we seeking to create a picture perfect ideal of ourselves that the world would find "Insta" worthy? As my mother used to say, "If everyone else was jumping off a bridge, would you do it too?" Perhaps it is time to stop soaking up so much social and print media and paying so much attention to what the world says about beauty and looks. Just because everyone else is obsessed with looks, size, and shape, doesn't mean we have to as well. We have a *choice*.

We were each fearfully and wonderfully created for a purpose. Figuring out what that purpose is and how we can best live it out is the journey of life. A healthy body and a mind free from bondage to thoughts guided by an internal critic help us do that. Remembering that the world is filled with propaganda and marketing gurus that want us to follow their worldly ways provides a guardrail for healthy living. Social and print media inform us about the trends of the day. Reminding ourselves that these are not barometers by which we are suppose to live provides another guardrail. They are not a mirror and lens from which we are to evaluate our self-worth.

In my own struggles with disordered eating and negative body image, I have found that knowing WHO and WHOSE I am has helped me keep my focus. Comparing myself with others only gets me off track. Remembering that God made people in all shapes, sizes, and colors, keeps me focused on truth. So whether you are pear shaped, oval, hourglass or a diamond shape, be the best version of you possible. Mindfully evaluate how you are doing. When you see you are falling into old habits, stop them in their tracks. When you realize the voice of your internal critic is getting louder, review the work you have done to quiet the voice. Repeat this process for another 40 days if necessary. Be the best YOU possible through nutrient rich foods and activity to keep you naturally feeling and looking your best. Live your best life in freedom and be all that God created you to be!

Appendix

We estimated how many session entry forms would be needed for each phase of the journey. If you run out of session journal entry space during any of the phases, you will find additional forms here. Please note that these are to be reproduced only for individual journaling purposes. These forms should not be reproduced for any other purpose.

If you don't want to reproduce these pages, feel free to use a notebook or other blank journal to write questions and answers for the additional days needed.

Phase One Session Log Sheet

Day 1 - Day 10

Complete the log for this food/exercise session. Place a checkmark next to or circle all that apply.

Date: **Day of Week:**   **Time:**   AM/PM

Reason for the session: Meal   Snack   Exercise   Other (Explain)

Who joined you: **Or Circle:**   Ate Alone/Exercised Alone

Did you count calories eaten or expended?   Yes   No   **Why?**

Meal/Snack location:

    Dining Table   Restaurant   In front of TV/Computer
    In bed   Automobile   Other (Explain)

Beverage Consumed:

    Soda   Diet soda/seltzer water   Tap/bottled water
    Milk/dairy alternative   Other (Explain)

Reason for Eating:

    Nourishment   Health   Social Activity/Group Gathering
    Coping with feelings   Controlling Emotions   Other (Explain)

Reason for Exercise: (Check or circle the major reasons)

    Appearance/Weight Maintenance   Fitness/Health Management
    Stress/Emotions/Mood or Feeling Management   Socializing

At the beginning, during, or conclusion of the meal/snack/exercise, I felt: (Circle all that apply to any phase of this session)

Bad	Numb	Panic	Empowered	Distressed	Successful
Worried	Anxious	Sad	Depressed	Relief	Motivated
Fear	Lonely	Angry	Contempt	Calm	Self-Disciplined
Comfort	Misery	Control	Driven	Soothed	Traumatized
Shame	Guilt	Tired	Hungry	Other (List)	

ACTIVITY REFLECTION

Journal some thoughts about the meal or snack you selected or the exercise you undertook. Why did you select what you did? How did the choices relate to the rules, habits, and rituals your internal critic helped you set up?

EMOTION REFLECTION

Journal about how the activity reflected the emotions you identified that went along with the activity. What brought the feelings/emotions on? Did they change during the session? What helped them change? Why did you select food/exercise as an outlet for those feelings?

**To be copied for additional session journaling.
Should not be reproduced for any other purpose.**

Phase Two Session Log Sheet

Day 11 - Day 20

Complete the log for this food/exercise session. Place a checkmark next to or circle all that apply.

Date: **Day of Week:** **Time:** AM/PM

Reason for the session: Meal Snack Exercise Other (Explain)

Meal/Snack location:

Dining Table	Restaurant	In front of TV/Computer
In bed	Automobile	Other (Explain)

Beverage Consumed:

Soda	Diet soda/seltzer water	Tap/bottled water
Milk/dairy alternative	Other (Explain)	

Reason for Eating:

Nourishment	Health	Social Activity/Group Gathering
Coping with feelings	Controlling Emotions	Other (Explain)

Exercise Location and Activity:

Who joined you: **Or Circle:** Ate Alone/Exercised Alone

Reason for Exercise: (Check or circle the major reasons)

Appearance	Fitness
Stress/Emotions/Mood	Socializing

Did you count calories eaten or expended? Yes No **Why?**

List feelings experienced before/during/after:

How did you respond to those feelings?

Did you think about using an alternative coping tool? Yes No

Did you use an alternative coping tool? If so, what did you do and what happened?

What positive steps did you take to apply self-control to your food/exercise habits, rituals, routines at this session?

Activity Reflection

Journal some thoughts about the meal or snack you selected or the exercise you undertook. Why did you select what you did? Did you have control of your rules, habits, and rituals or did they have control of you?

Emotion Reflection

Journal about the feelings you experienced and how you responded to them. Could you have taken a breath and considered an alternative option? If you did consider and select an alternative, what led you to do that? What allowed you to be more aware of your feelings and responses? If you did not consider an alternative option, what got in the way?

**To be copied for additional session journaling.
Should not be reproduced for any other purpose.**

Phase Three Session Log Sheet

Day 21 - Day 30

Complete the log for this food/exercise session. Place a checkmark next to or circle all that apply.

Date: **Day of Week:** **Time:** AM/PM

Reason for the session: Meal Snack Exercise Other (Explain)

Meal Components: Protein Fruit Whole grain Vegetable Healthy Fat

Method of Preparation:

Baked	Broiled	Sautéed	Grilled	Boiled
Fried	Roasted	Steamed	Stir-fry	Stewed
Fresh/raw	Frozen	Canned	Processed/packaged	
Prepared by others	Other (Explain)			

Beverage Consumed:

Soda Diet soda/seltzer water Tap/bottled water
Milk/dairy alternative Other (Explain)

Exercise Location and Activity:

Level of Activity: Easy Moderate Vigorous Highly Vigorous

Who joined you: **Or Circle:** Ate Alone/Exercised Alone

Feelings experienced before/during/after and how you responded to those feelings? Were they expressed in the session? If so, how and if not, why not?

What positive step did you take or guardrail did you apply during this session? Did it go as planned? Would you do anything differently next time?

Activity Reflection

Journal some thoughts about the meal or snack you selected or the exercise you undertook. How did the meal/snack look, smell, and taste? What did you notice going on around you as you exercised? How were you in control of this session and how did this session control you?

Emotion Reflection

Journal about the feelings you experienced and how you responded to them. Was this session a reflection of feelings and emotions? List some positive self-talk responses you can offer to your internal critic to combat the lies you hear in your head.

**To be copied for additional session journaling.
Should not be reproduced for any other purpose.**

Phase Four Session Log Sheet

Day 31- Day 40

Complete the log for this food/exercise session. Place a checkmark next to or circle all that apply.

Date:　　　　　　　　**Day of Week**:　　　　　　　　**Time**:　　　　　AM/PM

Reason for the session:　　Meal　　　　Snack　　　　Exercise　　　　Other (Explain)

Meal Components:　　Protein　　Fruit　　Whole grain　　Vegetable　　Healthy Fat

Method of Preparation:

Baked	Broiled	Sautéed	Grilled	Boiled
Fried	Roasted	Steamed	Stir-fry	Stewed
Fresh/raw	Frozen	Canned	Processed/packaged	
Prepared by others	Other (Explain)			

Beverage Consumed:

Soda	Diet soda/seltzer water	Tap/bottled water
Milk/dairy alternative	Other (Explain)	

Exercise Location and Activity:

Level of Activity:　　　　Easy　　　　Moderate　　　　Vigorous　　　　Highly Vigorous

Who joined you:　　　　　　　　**Or Circle**:　　　　Ate Alone/Exercised Alone

Journal about the session. Did past behaviors, situations, or emotional responses impact the session? How was this a nourishing session to your body? What positive steps did you take?

To be copied for additional session journaling.
Should not be reproduced for any other purpose.

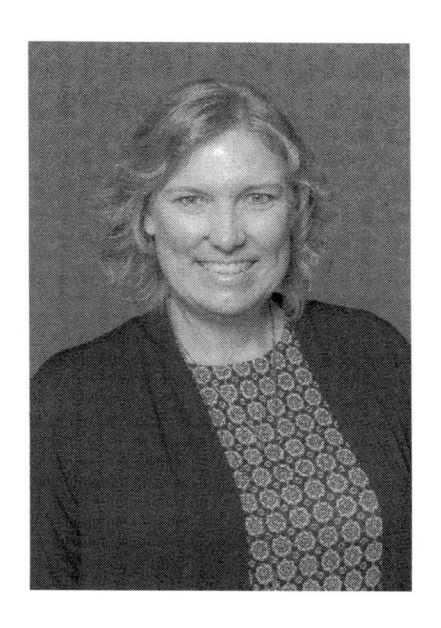

About the Author

Tanya Fasnacht Jolliffe, RDN, LD is a Registered Dietitian Nutritionist and Licensed Dietitian. She attended the College of Mount St. Joseph in Cincinnati, Ohio on a volleyball scholarship where she graduated with a Bachelor of Science degree in dietetics. After graduation, Tanya completed a dietetic internship and worked in several Cincinnati area hospitals, specializing in nutritional management of people with end-stage organ disease or solid organ transplant. Tanya has provided medical nutrition therapy and nutrition education in a variety of settings and has authored hundreds of educational articles and blogs. She has also presented as part of clinical teams, at seminars, and at conferences and expos.

Over the years, Tanya has been able to use her gifts and talents in a variety of ways such as leading discipleship classes for youth, and health promotion and risk reduction focused in the areas of transportation wellness and disordered eating. She has also been blessed to help companies and organizations develop program strategies to bring about growth. Tanya was recognized for her athletic success in high school by being inducted into the Greenville Senior High School Athletic Hall of Fame. It was icing on the cake when she was also recognized for success at the collegiate level and inducted into the Mount St. Joseph University Athletic Hall of

Fame. Tanya lives in the greater Cincinnati area of Ohio with her husband Scott. They are blessed to have their two grown children and their families living nearby.

Tanya's personal struggle with body image and disordered eating and exercise provided the framework for this project. Through the truth of God's word and His amazing grace, Tanya was able to see herself as God saw her and not as others told her she should be. Having been set free from worldly lies, she was able to embrace mindful eating and exercise practices and leave the disordered behaviors behind. Her prayer is that this journaling program will help other people find that same freedom.

Made in United States
Troutdale, OR
08/01/2023